PREGNANCY

the best state of the union

PREGNANCY

the best state of the union

by Waldo L. Fielding, M.D.

illustrations by Lawrence Duffy

The Bond Wheelwright Company
Publishers
Porter's Landing, Freeport, Maine

To *Suzanne, Jed,* and *Andy* —
No family can beat that union

And to *Paul,* who stated it all so well

Manufactured in the United States of America
Library of Congress Catalog Card No. 76-2152
ISBN 0-87027-147-4
Third, revised, printing of second edition

CONTENTS

LIST OF ILLUSTRATIONS

AN INTERESTING CONDITION

All right, so you're pregnant.

Wonderful!

But as you may have concluded as a result of unsolicited advice from all directions, it *has* happened before.

Over the countless centuries since women began to conceive, to grow their babies within themselves, and to deliver them, a sea of lore and legend has developed. And most of it is wrong. If you are pregnant for the first time, the chances are that you have already listened to more of this dubious history than you'd need for twelve babies.

Therefore, please remember this: old wives' tales are matched by myths earnestly told by young women, too. Both kinds represent the most subjective storytelling on earth.

Your sensible questions and your doctor's candid answers are the best possible guide through the fascinating biological process in which you have become involved.

The sole purpose of this book is to fortify you with the information you need to help you through the 267-odd days of your pregnancy so that you will know—now and at delivery time—exactly what you are doing.

And you'll know what your baby is doing, too.

If you are a practical woman you have probably already arranged for this inevitable event, or you will do so shortly. Over the course of the next several months the milestones of pregnancy will be marked in terms of the visits you will make to your doctor's office. Each of these visits will be increasingly important. They also will serve as convenient and logical divisions to estimate the growth of your baby and your adjustment to the fact of its ultimate birth.

An excellent way to manage your absorption of information about pregnancy, and a practical method of dividing a book about childbearing, is in terms of these monthly visits, with pertinent reference to the events to be expected as they occur. Therefore, as best as can be done, each section of this book contains what you need to know at the time you need to know it.

The most valuable medical information you can be given right now is that you are in a very normal, manageable condition known as pregnancy. Not "expectancy," not "in a family way," not "*enceinte.*" The bold, true and suitable word is "pregnant." Don't back away from it.

The overwhelming majority of pregnant women complete the process successfully. A great number of them have a wonderful time. Those who don't are missing a delightful experience which can easily be theirs. For in pregnancy, attitude can be everything, including the way you carry the bulge.

In this book I will try to emphasize the positive things a woman can do to improve her pregnancy and make it more fun, rather than compile a foreboding list of things she ought not to do. Pregnancy is an active process, not a passive one. Although much of it is pre-programmed by Nature, the carrier can still be the boss if she wants to be.

The woman who boldly puts herself in charge, even when not precisely sure of what she's doing, is the one who will derive pleasure, excitement and satisfaction from start to finish—not necessarily including the minor bumps along the way.

Most pregnancies are normal, but each of them is special. Quite naturally, *yours* is the baby you are most interested in at the moment. There are likely to be enough variations in your particular sequence of things over the coming months for you to know how special and different is your private gestation. There have been billions of babies born throughout history, but none of the mothers have had the same experience, and no one will be able to match yours.

So this book is intended to guide you through your special pregnancy, helping you to understand what to expect and to handle anything you don't expect. Your own good sense and the assistance of a physician you trust are all you need to make a smashing success of motherhood.

For a starter, let's make a pact: nothing that you will read in this book will vary significantly from what any competent, modern obstetrician regards as accepted current practice. This book is not an attempt to revolutionize the baby-bearing business.

For your part, please agree now not to be alarmed by anything you hear from Muriel or Mildred or Martha. They may have had a slew of babies, but they haven't had *yours.*

If you have any doubts about something you read in this book, ask your doctor. Take his advice even if that advice is to throw this book away!

Remember that we are living in the most rapidly paced period in history, with medicine far up among the front runners. Policies and practices which seemed inviolable ten years ago may already have been altered or discarded because of new knowledge.

This pace has a special application to obstetrics, because the field is as old as medicine itself. There's more tradition, lore and precedent in maternity care than in any other branch, and it tends to die hard. As a modern woman, you naturally want to deliver a modern baby under modern conditions. You will find much that is new in this book, but all of it has been carefully tested and researched. The advances promise you a healthier baby, less strain on yourself, and more confidence in going through the process.

So swift has been the pace of medical research that portions of this book had to be revised just before publication in order to take account of significant advances in obstetrical practice.

Women were once encouraged to bear their babies in ignorance. Doctors didn't want to upset their "delicate condition" with disturbing information. But we have since learned that there is nothing delicate about the condition of the normal pregnant woman. She's radiant with health and bursting with energy. She is also capable of understanding. To deny her information not only insults her, but forces her to fall back on ancient maternity lore that is notable more for its age than its accuracy.

There is nothing about your pregnancy that you should not know. But there is nothing about your pregnancy that you need to know too early. Therefore, let's take it one visit at a time, covering all of the miraculous and delightful changes that will occur as you accommodate the new person who has taken up residence within you.

This baby will make preposterous demands upon you. You will be astonished at your body's capacity to meet them.

This baby's first ultimatum is implicit in the very fact of its establishment within you: you must maintain the best possible level of health, since the baby is borrowing upon it. If you can also retain your good spirits despite the occasional strains and surprises, that's even better, and it will be greatly appreciated by your internal audience.

If you know what *you* are doing, and if you know what the *baby* is doing, then the two of you can make an excellent team.

And it couldn't matter less if it is only the two of you who appreciate how spectacular a pregnancy this one is going to be!

THE HAPPENING

You have more than a slight suspicion as to how you got pregnant in the first place. If the circumstance was special, you may even know when. Perhaps it will be interesting to know now just what happened internally.

Prevailing attitudes toward sex and love-making tend to downgrade a fact of rather staggering beauty: that from this simple and pleasurable union there can be produced an entirely new human being. There is nothing we know of in nature that is as dramatic, ingenious and impressive as the fact that each species contains the pattern and the material by which it can reproduce itself.

The wonder of it is conspicuous at the end of the process, for nobody is so sophisticated as to miss the uniqueness of her own baby. The beginning of the process is just as awesome for those who can consider it without inhibition.

For in conception, Nature is dealing with substances that are microscopic in their basic units. They are joined under conditions altogether beyond the conscious control of their donors. And they systematically and automatically begin to multiply themselves billions of times, until they finally emerge with hair like Mother's and a grin like Dad's.

And all that it takes is a man with sperm, a woman with an egg, and a place where the two cells can meet.

This is the simple biology that leads to conception. Only a single egg and a single sperm, each carrying its properly woven set of chromosomes, comprise the ultimate union. Precisely at the moment of conception one of every pair of the woman's chromosomes and one of every pair of the man's drops out of the action.

In joining, the two make up a new arrangement—half of hers matching half of his, pair for pair in exactly the correct order. Together they comprise a total plan for the construction of a baby. That plan includes the child's ultimate height, the color of its eyes, the placement of its tooth buds and—who knows—perhaps its response to an untuned violin.

The woman's contribution to this marvelous match parallels the contribution of her partner, with one major exception: She has nothing whatever to do with establishing the sex of the baby. The father alone determines that. It is his sperm that carries the extra chromosome which decides whether the new being is to be male or female.

At the time of conception there was a fantastic number of sperm—some four hundred million of them—vying for the chance to fertilize the ovum which was ready. About half carried the X chromosome, which could create a female offspring, and the other half bore the Y chromosome, which could only sponsor a boy.

From this fact you can draw a firm conclusion concerning the unknown sex of the baby: there is absolutely no basis, as far as we know, for a belief that boys "run" in your mother's family, or girls dominate on your husband's father's side. The sex of a child can neither be blamed upon nor credited to heredity. In the competitive race to reach the receptive ovum—and it *was* a race—there had to be a single winner out of the four hundred million, and the colts had no advantage over the fillies.

Several current investigators are exploring the possibilities suggested by an observable difference between male and female bearing sperm: the males swim faster, but the females endure longer. Therefore it is theorized that sperm arriving a day before or a day after the woman's egg is ready in the fallopian tube are somewhat more likely to be the slower but hardier female chromosome bearers.

But when the egg has been released close to the time of intercourse, more of the faster moving males may reach it first. So by timing the introduction of sperm relative to the time of ovulation, it is theoretically possible to favor whichever sex is desired.

However, experiments along these lines have been done mostly on bovine animals, so they do not yet have any practical application among humans.

There are also experiments being conducted by geneticists working with frozen sperm. They hope to isolate the sex chromosome under ultra-microscopy. When and if the method is perfected it may be possible to control the sex of artificially inseminated babies.

But most physicians—and most women, for that matter—feel that the mystery about which gender it is that is under development in the uterus is more interesting as a mystery than it would be as a question answered too early.

Suppose you could know, right now, whether you are carrying a girl or a boy, would it really matter? About the only significance of such knowledge is that it would tell you which color booties to work on, or suggest a motif for the bedroom that is to be done over.

You may fervently and actively hope for nine months that this baby will be a boy; but if it turns out that a girl is presented to you in the delivery room, you'll be delighted, and that's a promise. Anyone with experience in obstetrics will usually verify this axiom: no woman is disappointed by the sex of her baby, and most of them are delighted by it.

Though the gender of your baby remains a secret, there is not much mystery about the process which produced the internal climate necessary for the successful union of egg and sperm. It began with ovulation and climaxed with fertilization. Field conditions had to be perfect at the time.

In some animals—the rabbit, for instance—ovulation takes place when the female is stimulated by intercourse. But in the human female, ovulation takes place once each month with no relation to intercourse. Regular ovulation is a function of virgins, non-virgins, married and unmarried, and is based on the maturity of the female system. Each time, a single egg is released from either of the two ovaries.

There is a current suspicion that a phenomenon called supra-ovulation may also occur. This is the release of two eggs within a month, perhaps one from each ovary. Such a possibility would account for those rare instances when a woman produces two babies, each conceived at a different time, and perhaps delivered with a significant time interval between. But that is only a theory, and not much use to a woman who has enough to cope with knowing she now carries ONE egg that has been fertilized.

It happened within 48 hours of your last ovulation. Intercourse took place, all other internal conditions were favorable, and a sperm was able to fertilize the ovum.

No one knows yet how to tell exactly when a woman ovulates. Some clues can be found by examination of vaginal and cervical smears. Analyzing characteristics of the cervical mucus is a newer way of determining if ovulation has taken place. Fluctuations of body temperature from day to day give other hints. Signs are also found in studying samples of the tissue that lines the uterus—the endometrium .

Yet taken all together these indicators yield only a generality. We know that a woman is most likely to ovulate about 14 days before the start of her next menstrual period. The date of her previous period does not seem to have much influence.

So if a woman has a regular 28-day cycle, she can expect to ovulate on the 14th day. A woman with a 25-day cycle should ovulate on the 11th day—still 14 days before her next period.

This general rule is not likely to help much in any specific case. For the fact is that ovulation has been shown to occur, in one woman or another, on every single day of the cycle, including the days of menstruation.

If you now know that you are pregnant, the cycle no longer matters much. You ovulated under favorable conditions, sperm was available to fertilize the egg, and pregnancy was the result. Thus, with regular intercourse, a fairly normal cycle, and no preventive measures, conception is virtually inevitable.

When the egg was expelled from your ovary, it was swept directly into the fallopian tube. For a proper rendezvous to take place between egg and sperm, it must be in this tube, which is the only passageway to the uterus.

At the time the egg was released, your body had made further adjustments to be even more receptive. The cervical canal—the entrance into the uterus from the vagina—was filled with a transparent fluid that is hospitable and nourishing to spermatozoa and provides a medium through which they can swim toward their goal. Only once during the female cycle does this region become so tolerant; at other times the fluid is opaque and sticky, tending to impede and trap the sperm rather than assist them.

Although the optimum time for conception remains a mystery

for most women, there are some who know quite confidently when it arrives. They feel a special sort of pain—called *mittelschmertz*—which is sensed at the site of the ovary at the moment the egg is forced out. There may also be a slight discharge from the vagina.

Women who experience these signs are rare—and lucky—for they can achieve or avoid pregnancy accordingly. If such signals were more often noticeable among women the practice of the rhythm method of birth control would be far more successful. But most women know only what they learn from the calendar and their past experience with the menstrual cycle.

Those who have difficulty in conceiving may ask why, with so many million sperm available, can't at least a few reach the waiting egg?

The hazards to sperm are formidable. When they are ejaculated into the upper vagina, some will swim directly toward the cervix, which is their most promising avenue. But most are trapped in the vagina, whose slightly acid medium destroys them.

Those that enter the cervical canal are aided by the fluid there, which becomes alkaline only during the time of the cycle when an ovum is ready. This fluid not only protects the sperm but nourishes them as they continue on through the uterus and into the fallopian tubes.

This is a hazardous and arduous journey for the microscopic, short-lived sperm. It is estimated that an individual sperm can advance about one inch in eight minutes. But this is a random trip, never in a straight line. About half of the competitors will enter the wrong fallopian tube, if it happens to be the other that has received the egg from its ovary that month. So, of the comparative few that survive by passing through the cervix, the number again is drastically reduced.

Of the original 400 million, perhaps some 2,000 sperm will reach the site in the proper tube where the receptive egg is waiting. These 2,000 have traversed the cervix, then negotiated the two inches or so of the sea within the uterus, and finally struggled up half the length of the tube or more.

At the end of their journey, only one of them can fertilize the egg. What is the element of luck that determines the winner, and how are the also-rans disposed of? We don't know yet. But we can estimate broadly that it takes 30 to 45 minutes from the time of entry until the event of mating takes place. If an ovum has not yet arrived in the fallopian tube, it is believed that the eligible sperm can remain active and viable there for as long as 60 to 72 hours.

Nature allows a smaller margin of time for the ovum. If ovulation has taken place before intercourse, the egg will only remain healthy and receptive in the fallopian tube for a few hours. Then it will deteriorate, fragment and become ready for disposal.

This disparity of survival time complicates the problem of determining when the conception actually took place. Not only is it difficult to establish when ovulation occurred, but it is virtually impossible to determine if the fertilizing sperm was deposited that day, or at a time before or after.

In order to complete the genetic union, the sperm must first penetrate the egg's outer coating. To do this, the sperm is equipped with a special chemical called hyaluronidase. The necessity of softening the egg's covering may be one reason why so many hundreds of sperm are in the neighborhood. Still completely unknown is how one lone sperm manages the entry, barring all others; how much its swimming motion assists, and whether it takes advantage of the softening action supplied by other sperm in order to break through.

But once that sperm has made its entry its nucleus immediately combines with that of the egg, all other contestants are ruled out, and fertilization is complete.

Immediately the wondrous process of reproduction begins; the chromosome chains are matched, the unwanted material is rejected, and growth begins. The fertilized egg divides from one cell into two, then into four, then sixteen, squaring its number with each division until there are thousands, millions and ultimately billions of cells that comprise the full-term baby.

Though all of these cells begin in exactly the same way, some have special destinies. Some harden into bone, some group to form organs such as heart and lungs, and some become blood cells to flow through those that have formed themselves into vessels. Intertwined in each double helix of each cell is the code that tells the cell where to locate, when enough of a certain tissue has been produced, and how to repair and replace parts as needed.

Such is the baffling, wonder-filled sequence which, if you are pregnant, has already begun within your body.

The newly fertilized egg continues its gentle journey down the fallopian tube into the uterus, where most of its growth will take place. The trip takes six to seven days, during which time the subtle process of cell division continues. By the time the tiny passenger enters the spacious uterus, its total count of body cells still numbers less than 100.

After entering the uterus, the miniature baby-to-be floats around in the sea of fluid for a period of one to three days. Then it somehow finds a suitable place on the uterine wall, implants itself there, and settles down to the inexorable process of becoming an infant human.

By the 12th day, growth has become vigorous and certain. Yet the woman within whom all this impressive action has taken place has not yet missed her first menstrual period, and in all likelihood has no suspicion that she is pregnant.

YES, MY DEAR...

An event as regular and interruptive as menstruation cannot be ignored when it occurs. This is just about as true when it doesn't. With each day of lateness, suspicion increases until a stark decision must be made: pretend that nothing has happened, or find out if it has. A professional medical finding must be made, and if conception is verified, a program of care must begin.

You need a doctor.

And not just *any* doctor, for this one is to become increasingly important to you over the coming months. By the time you are ready to deliver you may come to regard this physician as the third most important person in your life, granting priority to the baby inside you and the partner who helped plant it there.

You will do well to make your choice with utmost care.

There are two kinds of physicians from which to choose: the general practitioner whose work includes the delivery of babies; and the specialist who is specifically trained in obstetrics.

The obstetrician's fee may be higher, but you can measure with this his study and experience in the field of medicine that now directly affects you and your baby.

Consider too that most pregnancies go along without major problems. If complications occur, the general practitioner will recognize them and probably suggest consultation. When the care of a specialist becomes necessary, the original consideration of fees will be academic, for the combined cost will be just about the same as for having an obstetrician over the entire pregnancy.

The choice of physician is your prime decision to make, and you ought to make it now; for even as you have been reading, your baby has continued to grow.

At least as important as fee and training is the doctor's personality. He must be one with whom you feel at ease. He must inspire your confidence rather than your awe. He ought to give you the feeling that he is giving you all the time you need and that he welcomes any questions you ask.

Peace of mind in pregnancy can be as important as diet or weight. The doctor you select ought to be one from whom you sense an immediate arm of support.

Therefore choose carefully; his importance to you will increase in direct proportion to the increase in size of your baby.

Friends who have had babies are likely to rave about the doctor who attended them. That's fine, for it means they chose well for themselves. This does not mean, however, that they would choose as wisely for you.

They may have chosen their doctor because he happened to be in vogue at the moment, or because his approach and personality appealed to them. Listen to them, of course, but temper their advice with that of a doctor whom you know. A physician's reputation among his colleagues is a dependable guide. It's a good bet that a family doctor who knows you can select someone about whom *you* may later choose to rave.

But suppose you happen to be brand new to your community, with every doctor in town a stranger? The local medical society can offer a list of qualified men with details of their background and training. In making your choice, there is no need to hesitate about asking questions. A physician is a scientist; he will respect your own intelligent research. He may be the most popular man around, but remember this: it is *you* who are carrying the baby, and *he* will carry the responsibility of helping you to deliver it.

Most women have hundreds of questions to ask as pregnancy advances. Each month of development produces its special sensations, and each of the dozen or so prenatal visits becomes an increasingly important event. Ideally, these visits should build toward such rapport between patient and doctor that she can enter the hospital absolutely confident that she and her medical ally are committed to her successful delivery.

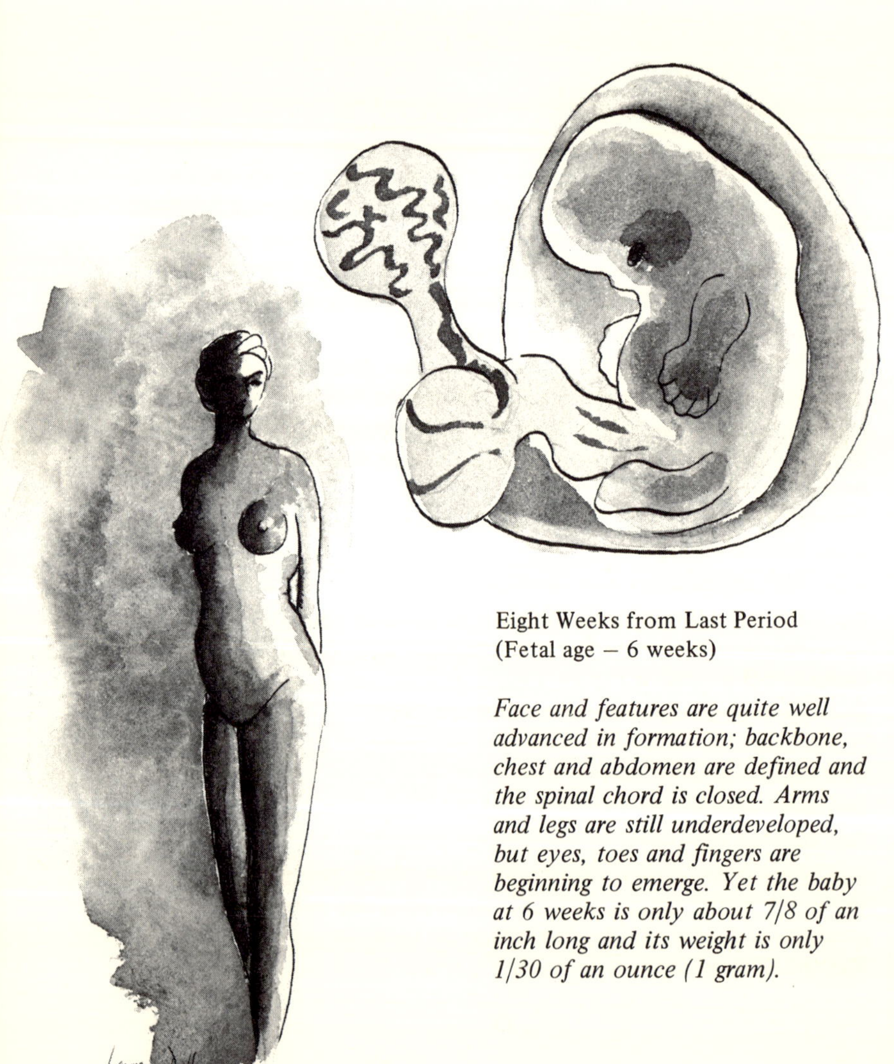

Eight Weeks from Last Period
(Fetal age — 6 weeks)

Face and features are quite well advanced in formation; backbone, chest and abdomen are defined and the spinal chord is closed. Arms and legs are still underdeveloped, but eyes, toes and fingers are beginning to emerge. Yet the baby at 6 weeks is only about 7/8 of an inch long and its weight is only 1/30 of an ounce (1 gram).

FIRST OFFICE VISIT
IN THE SECOND MONTH

circumstantial evidence

When a woman misses her second period, she is likely to consider pregnancy as more than a slight possibility. Establishing proof has now become so simple that it is most often done before actually seeing the doctor.

Usually, when a woman telephones a doctor's office for an appointment concerning pregnancy, she will routinely be sent first to a laboratory, where she gives a specimen of her urine. The specimen is tested to determine the presence of a hormone that is not normally present unless conception has occurred. By itself a positive test doesn't "prove" pregnancy, but along with the absence of periods, it's pretty dependable evidence.

The telltale hormone is called chorionic gonadotrophin. (Term-droppers, make the most of it.)

A newer test has been developed that takes only three minutes to complete. But until it becomes more reliable, most women agree that there's no rush; pregnancy lasts a good long while.

Assuming, then, that most women arrive at the doctor's office with their pregnancy already confirmed, what comes next? Usually it is the rather jolting announcement that they are not quite as pregnant as they thought they were.

This is because a woman who has missed two periods is only about six weeks along rather than eight. For she was obviously not pregnant at the time of her last period. It took about two weeks from that time for an ovum to be made ready and for internal conditions to become favorable for conception. It was intercourse at that time which resulted in fertilization. The urine test after the second missed period verified a suspicion that probably began to arise after the first missed period. The event that interrupted the cycle took place about two weeks before that.

When the first visit opens with pregnancy firmly established, the doctor begins by taking a comprehensive history, for nearly everything in a woman's physical life, past and present, has a bearing upon her condition.

This is true because the entire body is involved in the process of pregnancy, including the scars it may have accumulated, the diseases it has weathered, and the general level of health. Questions that may seem remote key the doctor to possibilities which must be taken into account.

But because of the nature of maternity, the term "history" can be misleading. One patient got the wrong idea altogether when told her history would have to be taken. She said, "But those are things I wouldn't tell *any*one!"

In the case of a newcomer to pregnancy, just about nothing is known concerning her capability of carrying and delivering a baby. Thus everything about her, medically and psychologically, is of importance to the doctor. Childhood diseases indicate what immunities she carries; scars, past surgery and once-broken limbs suggest special considerations in her management.

A childhood illness that may have affected the heart must be most carefully evaluated. If there is diabetes in the family, its manifestation in the woman must be guarded against. A past liver ailment, history of asthma, or a seasonal allergy—all these could complicate a pregnancy, which is why the doctor must know about them at the beginning.

The patient who takes a little time to organize this medical record before visiting the doctor will find him all smiles as she recites it.

It will make a significant difference whether this is a first pregnancy. If a woman has delivered a good-sized baby with no particular difficulty, then the doctor will know she has an adequate pelvis through which another large baby can pass. But if the first baby was small, he will be concerned about whether a larger one can negotiate the pelvis.

The length of time required for past labor, how difficult or easy it was, and the reaction to the medication and anesthesia used also guide the doctor in his special plans for the patient.

After all these questions about your medical past, you'll get down to the nitty-gritty: Was it difficult for you to conceive? Were you taking the contraceptive pill? When did you first menstruate as a girl? How regular are your periods, and how long do they last?

A doctor can even learn something about you from noting whether you refer to your periods as "the curse" or "my friend."

The doctor will be very interested to know whether you have had pain or discomfort during your periods. If you have lived with monthly cramps for years, take heart, for there is a possible consolation for you at the time of labor and delivery. Women whose periods are accompanied by cramps very often have a high threshold for labor contractions. Sometimes we find women whose periods have been a monthly endurance trial who say that labor is a breeze by comparison to the cramps they have had to tolerate.

If your periods included the symptoms of swollen hands and feet, you may find that the doctor will be especially stern about your weight control. There is a possible relationship between swelling—caused by fluid retention—and a complication of late pregnancy called toxemia of pregnancy. This is a condition that can be anticipated and controlled, especially if the patient tips the doctor ahead of time.

These are some of the questions the doctor will ask. There may be many others, depending on how you answer.

But your big question—the one that has top priority with most women—that's the hard one to answer.

When am I going to deliver?

Your approximate due date is calculated from the first day of your last period, according to Naegele's Rule. Dr. Naegele was a fine obstetrician, but his guideline works only as well as a patient's recollection of her last period.

You count back three months from the start of the last period, add seven to ten days, and hope you come up with a birthday. For example, if the start of the last period came on June 1, the E. D. C. (Estimated Date of Confinement) would be March 8 to March 11.

Though this system is far from a shot in the dark, it may be a little like changing a fuse by the light of a candle. Most women deliver between 39 and 41 weeks after the start of their last menstrual period. You probably will, too.

If your cycles have usually been short, be ready ahead of time. Women with long cycles are somewhat likely to find themselves sitting around for a few extra days.

Nothing else seems to affect the time of delivery. It doesn't change with age; race has no influence, nor how many times a woman has been pregnant, nor her physical size. There is a nonmedical rule that a baby will choose to be born at the least convenient and most unexpected time. You may include this maxim in your plans for your final week, but don't be surprised if the baby manages to thwart you anyway.

Another basis for working out a delivery date is to count 267 days forward from the time of conception. A woman who has been keeping fairly precise records for the purpose of intentional conception will have a good set of figures to start with. If she's a dropout from the rhythm method, she may know even better. When there happens to be an isolated incident of intercourse, then there will be little doubt.

Sometimes a doctor picks up some fairly interesting incidental information while a woman is trying to pinpoint the date of conception: "Let's see—Harry's mother was here for the weekend, so it must have been that Monday." Or, "I remember—right after his Milwaukee trip."

Then there is the happily married woman who may smile coyly and say, "I haven't the faintest idea."

But most often the date of conception is hazy at best. Later, when a woman feels the first movement of the baby inside her, she may start doodling with the calendar again, for there is another rule that says the baby will be born 19 weeks later. But this can just as likely be 18 weeks or 20 weeks, offering 14 days to guess at, which is no better than the odds Naegele offers. In fact, with a first pregnancy, early fetal movements can be so subtle that they are misinterpreted or missed altogether.

Therefore, how about this for a compromise: you are going to have a baby—sometime. Count on the baby to let you know when.

A question the doctor will ask—possibly in a deliberately casual manner—is whether there have been twins in either family. He is not necessarily hinting at a surprise, glad or otherwise. The question is important because the size of the uterus is a clue to the current stage of the pregnancy; if the uterus happens to be unusually large at this stage, multiple birth is a possible reason.

Twins used to occur once in about every 88 pregnancies. The square of that figure, around 7,500, was the average for triplets, and the cube, about 700,000, covered quadruplets. Actually these odds have changed with the advent of pills that can cause a non-ovulating woman to ovulate. Because dosage has not yet been accurately determined, a woman on certain pills may produce multiple births, may release more than one egg at a time. Ironically, these pills sometimes cause as many as 7 to 8 fetuses—which cannot possibly survive in the human uterus, and the pregnancy terminates in miscarriage long before maturity takes place. If you've been dreaming about a matched set of five whose life story can be sold to a magazine, forget it; you're still working against odds of around 60 million to one.

The majority of multiple births occur in women who are between the ages of 20 and 45. A tendency toward twin-bearing is hereditary, and is carried by the male and female equally. Twins do not necessarily skip a generation as the legend promises, so if there are such pairs in your family and in your husband's, too, keep an eye out for a good deal on a two-place perambulator.

I had one patient to whom I had been hinting the possibility of a multiple birth, and who was not at all delighted at the prospect. Ultimately I sent her over for an X-ray to verify my guess. I got a call from the X-ray man, who said, "Would you believe it: She hasn't got two in there, she's got *three!*"

Knowing her alarm, I told him not to tell her anything, but to put the X-rays in an envelope and send her back with them. She came in with her husband and her other two children. I put the X-ray print up on a view-box and said to her, "There, you see, my dear, I was right."

She released a little sigh of resignation. Then I pointed to one head with a pencil and said, "There's *one* baby."

One sob.

"And there's another baby."

Two sobs.

At this point I had my arm around her for security, then I said, "And see, down here, there's a *third* baby!"

And she let out, in a wail, "Oh! I'll be the only Jewish mother in the world who has so many children!"

I must include the outcome of this story, even though it doesn't have the slightest pertinence here:

I alerted the hospital that we could expect triplets on the anticipated date, and special arrangements were made, for such a birth is a big event. All three shifts of nurses rehearsed their roles, and extra incubators were provided.

It happened that the woman went into labor just about when expected, and called me. I sent her along, then called the hospital myself. Such was the state of readiness that I knew that all I had to say was, "She's on her way!"

The nurse who answered gave me the least likely response of all possible responses under all possible conditions:

"Oh?" she said coolly, "*Another* set of triplets?"

My patient's babies were born consecutively following another set delivered as a complete surprise by a woman who had walked in, unanticipated. I have since been told that the odds against consecutive sets of triplets are 59 million to one!

Eventually all doctors run out of questions and arrive at the time for the physical examination. You will be weighed and measured for height. If necessary, a sample of urine will be taken to verify pregnancy. A blood sample will be drawn for determination of blood type, Rh factor and level of red cells. Most states also require that a pregnancy examination include testing the blood for syphilis.

The doctor will also record blood pressure, pulse, heartbeat and chest sounds.

Your breasts will be very carefully examined, as should always be the case in a thorough workup of a mature woman. If you plan to breast feed, the doctor may recommend that you get started on daily soap-and-water scrubbings to toughen the nipple area.

After this general examination of your body, the doctor will ask you to mount the rather stark table whose purpose you have understood and perhaps dreaded all along. You are about to have a pelvic examination, and if it's your first, you may regard the prospect as the ultimate humiliation of womanhood.

It is nothing of the kind, of course. Even so, every woman has one attitude or another toward it, and those stirrups don't help. But a pelvic examination is really not so bad, and it is enormously informative to the doctor.

If the uterus has changed from its small, firm pear shape to one that is soft, doughy and enlarged, this tends to confirm pregnancy. The examination will also determine whether you have a small pelvis or a large one. Nothing ominous is suggested by the finding that the pelvic capacity is modest, for such women usually have small babies. Remember that Nature is the boss here, and she likes to do her work neatly, matching baby to mother compatibly in better than 95 per cent of her cases. Her occasional lapses are what obstetricians are for.

An instrument the doctor will use is called a speculum. These days most of them are made of disposable plastic. The speculum enables the doctor to look for a slight bluish tinge to the vagina and cervix, a dependable indication that the changes that follow conception are taking place. The instrument also allows us to do the Pap smear for cancer detection and one for gonorrhea if requested or considered advisable.

Information obtained from the doctor during this examination sometimes inspires a woman's resolve to exercise conscious control over the size of her baby. If told she has a small pelvis, she may determine to eat cautiously so as not to produce a big baby. She may elect to eat heartily on the theory that she will thus produce a more robust infant. Either approach is quite futile, for a baby's size is pretty much pre-programmed. A skimpy diet might produce a slightly smaller baby, but a heavy diet will not produce a bigger one.

The major weight concern is how heavy the mother is. When a doctor finds a patient already overweight he is likely to be quite stern about having her cut down on intake. A woman whose weight matches her build ought to follow a normal, nutritious diet. Very few women are advised to eat heartily even though they may be a few pounds underweight at the outset of pregnancy.

The standard generally followed is that a woman should not gain more than 20 pounds over her entire term. This is probably the most important assignment of pregnancy, almost always difficult to follow. Can you do it?

There may be temptation from recent national publicity given to the claim that most doctors don't let their patients gain enough weight during pregnancy. The 20-pound-maximum rule is being challenged on

the grounds that a greater margin of weight increase ought to be allowed to insure optimum growth of the baby and reserve for the mother to
draw upon after delivery. But so far as I am concerned, and I think this
is true of most obstetricians, the hazards of excessive weight gain are far
more menacing than any disadvantages that might be shown by further
research in having a woman go to term while adhering to the 20-pound
rule. Ultimately it may become possible to compute to the ounce how
much weight any given woman ought to gain in her pregnancy. But
until then, we must respect the fact that weight control remains a
difficult problem of pregnancy and requires continued discipline by the
woman. She must keep her weight down.

One of the simplest ways to do it is to eliminate from the diet a
group of foods best known as the Fattening Four: bread, butter,
potatoes and dessert. A sensible resolve of pregnancy is to give up the
Fattening Four the moment you know you are pregnant.

As for the positive aspect of diet, that is quite flexible. You don't
have to down extra milk as women did in former days, because the
vitamin and mineral supplements you'll be taking will insure that you're
getting all the nutrients you and your baby require.

And just as you may eat normally, except for the Fattening Four,
so may you live normally, too. If you have a job and would like to
continue working, go ahead, right up until labor starts, if nobody
objects. If you're running a home, there's no need for a radical change
in routine.

All that pregnancy requires is sensible consideration of an altered
condition; it does not demand that a woman drop everything for nine
months to sit around and think beautiful thoughts.

One of the lingering bugaboos is travel: women formerly were
told never to take any major trips. This is silly. You may go wherever
you like, with only minor consideration of your condition. Take along
a list of medical way-stations so you'll know where to go for help if you
need it.

As for activity, you may play tennis, ride a bicycle, swim, bowl,
or spin a hoop around your waist. And if you can manage that last one
in your eighth month, you're a pretty good bet for a TV show.

The sensible precautions about activity are these: quit when you
feel tired, and stick to the functions for which your body has already

had some training. A new sport or skill might demand stresses and strains for which your altered anatomy is not well prepared.

But DON'T ski, no matter how good you are. It's not that you might hurt the baby, you might break a leg, which would be a dreadful inconvenience in late pregnancy. You may want to knit booties, but certainly not bones.

How about sexual intercourse during pregnancy?

Why not?

Love doesn't stop just because a woman is gestating, so neither must love-making.

Some doctors think that a woman ought to refrain from sex on those days that she would normally be having a period, on the chance that she might be more vulnerable to miscarriage then. This has not been shown to be medically valid, but most miscarriages do occur at the time of the second or third missed period. So although we are not sure that the uterus is more irritable at these times it may be wise to refrain from intercourse.

If intercourse is comfortable and pleasurable, carry on. You may want to do some shifting of position as your center of balance changes and as your buige becomes bulgier. Most doctors advise their patients to refrain late in pregnancy, but that time is still several months away.

Smoke if you must, but moderately. In spite of all the evidence that smoking damages the body, people insist on continuing, and pregnant women are not an exemplary exception. But if you can cut down, or if you can use pregnancy as motivation to quit altogether, you will obviously improve your physical condition. New research suggests that heavy smoking may be related to premature delivery, which surely ought to be an incentive to cut down or quit.

As for alcohol, drink if you must, but take it easy. Heavy drinking could very well hurt the baby, could cause mental retardation. And any pregnant woman, tipsy, is remembered by too many people. Why not classify a third cocktail under "dessert," which you can't have anyway?

Currently in vogue is the practice of joining a prenatal exercise group for the purpose of toning up the body so it can carry and deliver with optimum efficiency. Such training is fine if the woman enjoys it and feels she is deriving benefit. But there's not much point for her to take part only because she thinks she ought to. Women sometimes feel that carrying a baby requires them to become instant athletes, and they go at it with such fervor that they become clusters of sore muscles.

If group exercise doesn't happen to appeal to you, there's no need to feel guilty about it.

There's a good possibility, however, that activity within a group of women who are also pregnant might be enjoyable. There is no question about the benefits of well-directed exercise for anyone's body. But don't expect that it will guarantee a delivery that is so free of strain that you can pluck your eyebrows while it's going on.

Your doctor will probably encourage any physical activity that improves your general health, but check out any special endeavor with him to be sure. It is doubtful that he'll encourage scuba diving or bouncing on a trampoline, but you'll find him quite reasonable about most things you might want to do.

In fact, in your first interview, many more of your questions are likely to be answered, "yes" than you may have expected.

There is one firm, inflexible "no." You may NOT take any kind of medication, pill, powder, tablet or shot without specific clearance from the doctor. It is impossible for a pregnant woman to take something for herself without also taking it for the baby, on whom it may have a dangerous effect. Therefore all medications, including those routinely taken before pregnancy, must be taken only with the doctor's approval.

One thing the doctor may give you, then and there, is a polio booster, even though you probably have had the Salk or Sabin series in the past.

We don't fool around with polio as a possibility in pregnancy. Just about every sensible physician anywhere will verify a pregnant woman's polio vaccine status and reinforce her with an oral booster. The longevity of immunization is not yet precisely known. It has been firmly established, however, that there is no danger in receiving an annual booster, so my patients usually get one. Even if it is ultimately proved a useless precaution, many of us will regard it as a solemn ritual toast to one of the truly great conquests over disease in the history of medicine.

You will learn during your first visit that your doctor expects the relationship between the two of you to consist of more than monthly visits leading up to labor and delivery. He wants to hear from you whenever anything unusual occurs. One sign which means a woman *must* contact her doctor is bleeding. Any show of blood in pregnancy must be evaluated.

In the stage between six and ten weeks there can be a minor bleeding event associated with implantation. What happens is that the fertilized egg seeks destination and security as it floats around in the amniotic fluid of the uterus. When it comes into contact with a suitable site on the uterine wall it actually burrows in, sometimes eroding through a few small blood vessels. This is the source of the sparse and brief implantation bleeding.

Unfortunately, such bleeding is difficult to distinguish from a kind that may indicate a threat of miscarriage. Generally, implantation bleeding is not accompanied by cramps, as is an attempt to miscarry. Implantationbleeding does not increase, and it usually stops in two or three days, which further assures the doctor that miscarriage is not impending.

Psychologically, this may seem a poor time to mention the possibility of miscarriage, especially to readers who are pregnant for the first time. But it is important that every woman understand a basic fact about her female system:

If a woman miscarries during her first three months of pregnancy, the probabilities are very high that she does not lose a baby; rather, she loses an imperfect egg (a blighted ovum). Such a miscarriage is the correction of an error by the body.

Perhaps the egg was slightly past its prime, making the conception imperfect; or the internal "climate" was not ideal to sustain the fertilized egg. Nature thus protects the woman by spontaneous abortion, rejecting an imperfect product. Her body is spared from useless strain and she avoids the disappointment of a fruitless pregnancy.

The distinction contains a comfort: it is easier to accept the disappointment of a faulty conception than to accept the loss of a baby. No baby was lost; only an opportunity.

Here is the supporting evidence of this assertion: some ten per cent of all pregnancies end in miscarriages. At least half of these are so structurally imperfect that they could not have developed into a being.

Therefore it makes sense to accept a tenet that most obstetricians believe: if what you have inside you is suited to develop into a complete baby, your body will allow it to do so. If not, Nature will usually bail you out.

But what about accidents—a fall down the stairs, an auto collision, a blow to the abdomen from a swinging door? Don't worry about such events. If you have a firmly established pregnancy in your uterus it is just about as stable as any organ in your body. Even a sharp, powerful assault directly over the site is not likely to dislodge a normally implanted baby, because that baby has become a part of your body, no more vulnerable than any other part. In cases where a miscarriage does occur following an accident, the miscarriage was probably inevitable anyway.

Because the benevolent aspect of miscarriage in cases of blighted ovum is not well understood, a woman who shows signs of an impending rejection may want treatment to prevent it. This is almost always discouraged. It is true that certain hormones may decrease the body's attempts to miscarry. But if what the uterus contains is not destined to become a baby, it obviously ought not to be retained.

Rarely, there are exceptions. When a doctor sees a woman with a history of several miscarriages and finds other evidence that she may be losing normal pregnancies, he might try to help her to retain the baby by giving her hormones. But most often the difficulty of continuing a sound conception will not manifest itself until after three months. That is when the doctor can use hormones with greater confidence that they may be a means to continue what, by that time, is a firmly established pregnancy.

Benevolent percentages suggest that, even at six weeks or so, yours is already a firmly established pregnancy. What does a baby look like at that state of development? It's fairly impressive for so short a time. Face and features are quite well advanced in formation; backbone, chest and abdomen are defined and the spinal cord is closed. Arms and legs are still underdeveloped, but eyes, toes and fingers are beginning to emerge. Yet a fetus at six weeks is only about seven-eighths of an inch long.

Such a baby doesn't take up much space yet, but it will. The uterus will have to expand over 500 times its normal size to accommodate it. (The mother doesn't get quite that big, although she may feel that she does.)

If all of this sounds breezy and uncomplicated, you may be tempted to conclude with some cynicism that most obstetricians are men, very few of whom find themselves pregnant. It is only fair and realistic, therefore, to deal with those phases of the process that are not so rosy.

For example, consider the traditional term "morning sickness."

Newly pregnant women are often distressed to discover that the nausea of the first trimester can overtake them any time of day. Fortunately there is now quite a battery of pills to control and eliminate this discomfort.

There is also a non-pill cure that can be highly effective: abandon the ill-founded notion that unless you get sick, you're not really pregnant. The fact happens to be that plenty of women sail through their first three months with no such upsets or discomforts. There are surely others whose queasiness is caused more by an idea in the mind than by a chemical change in the body.

Whatever is the cause, there is no reason to suffer in silence in the belief that nausea is a necessary ingredient of pregnancy. The doctor can help find the medication that is most effective. He may also help his patient uncover any hidden reason that is intensifying her discomfort. In any case, the condition will almost always correct itself around the end of the third month.

What about some of the weird cravings that are said to come over expectant women? If you don't have any, don't be disappointed. If there ever was any validity to the old pickles-and-ice-cream story it probably derived from the fact that in some cultures the diet wasn't very good, and women unconsciously sought to supplement it with foods containing the necessary baby-building materials. There are impoverished places in America, for example, where pregnant women suck mouthfuls of a certain kind of clay.

Another explanation for cravings may be that they arise because of the necessary strictness in weight control. A hungry woman naturally thinks about food, including dishes she may never have tried. And of course, some women have special cravings in pregnancy solely because they think the pregnancy would be incomplete without them.

I don't see much possible harm here; in fact, indulging an odd craving can often be fun. A most sensible Boston woman nibbled ice cubes through all eight of her pregnancies and had a marvelous time—she even used to bring her own tray of miniature cubes to parties.

There's a reverse side to this phenomenon, too. You may experience a sudden, strong dislike for a favored food, or for smoking, or for odors that have never been offensive to you before. These strange aversions are often startling when they occur, but it is pointless to stew over them. Pregnancy entitles you to privileges, so take what you can get. There is no guarantee, however, that the flow of sympathy will be so abundant that your husband will be ready to dash out into the snow at 3:45 *a. m.* to find a place that sells hot knockwurst and sauerkraut.

An oddity of early pregnancy that is strictly physical is drowsiness; it may suddenly overtake you in the early weeks. Some women find that they seem to tire almost instantly when they try to work. They often feel that they'd like to sleep through most of the day. If your position at home makes extra sleep possible, go ahead, and don't let guilt spoil your naps.

But if you have responsibilities—a job, or other children—be assured that forcing yourself to get busy will dispel the sleepy feeling in short order.

For a woman who has several small children to tend, a husband to feed, and a house to maintain, there is a sound medical explanation for the deep fatigue felt at bedtime:

She's tired!

Another common annoyance of early pregnancy is the frequent need to urinate. This is nothing more than a nuisance and it has no other cure but time. The cause is the enlarging uterus pressing on the bladder, making you feel more acutely the normal signal that it is time for relief. After a few weeks the uterus will rise up out of the pelvis, taking most of its pressure off the bladder.

Later, toward delivery time, the baby will move down into the lower pelvis, and you'll find yourself checking the location of powder rooms again.

If there have been any other discomforts or strange sensations in the early days of pregnancy they ought to be mentioned in the first visit, no matter how odd you may think them to be. A woman expecting a baby is as entitled to reassurance as she is to medication, and her doctor will be glad to give it.

Besides, it is entirely possible that *he* may be writing a book, too, and so may be able to use the story.

The first visit will probably end with the doctor loading you down with a fair amount of homework. He'll have booklets, weight charts, diet suggestions and pamphlets to help you expand your knowledge of the pregnancy process.

You'll find most of this material fairly fascinating, no matter how sophisticated you may think you are, for pregnancy is the most spectacular personal business to which any woman can attend.

Even if you have had four or five children, read the material anyway; it will provide a few well-merited laughs, along with some pleasant sentimental recollections. Besides, there probably are several new wrinkles since your last HURRAH—!

By the end of this lengthy first visit, you and the doctor are probably in tune. He has confirmed your condition, given you an estimated date of confinement, and answered most of your questions.

Now he becomes your partner in an exciting venture—the production of a baby who will be altogether special among humankind, simply because it is yours.

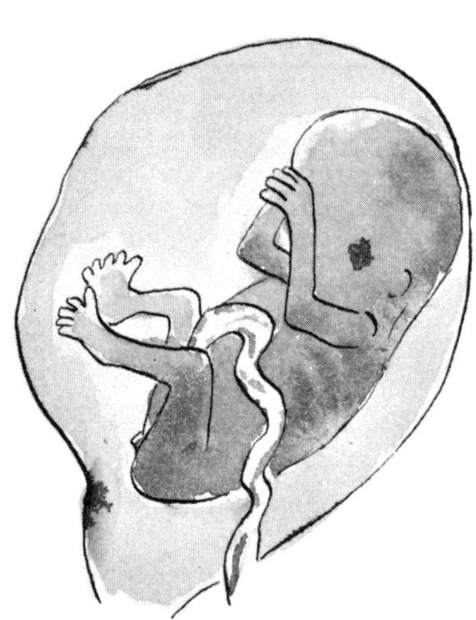

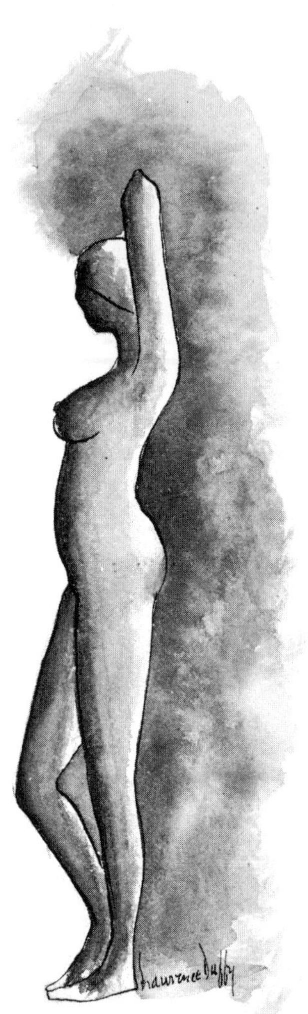

Twelve Weeks from Last Period
(Baby's age — 10 weeks)

*Measures slightly over 3 inches
in length and weighs about 1 ounce.
The sex is indistinguishable. Fingers and toes are differentiated,
and nails are beginning to appear.
The kidneys are now making urine,
which escapes into the amniotic
fluid. The baby moves but the
movements are too weak to be
felt by the mother.*

SECOND OFFICE VISIT
IN THE THIRD MONTH

who's that with you?

By the time of the second office visit, a month later, you will have missed your third period. With luck you may also have had time enough to persuade your husband to come to the doctor's office with you.

After all, pregnancy started out as a family affair and ought to continue that way.

For far too long, pregnancy has been considered the woman's domain alone. Husbands have remained as aloof as possible, and even if they happen to display some concern for what's going on, doctors and hospitals tended to shunt them aside.

Now, at long last, we are beginning to respect the obvious fact that maternity is the man's business, too. This is why I welcome the husband at the second visit, and hope to keep him informed all along the way.

As for hospital policy, more and more institutions are coming to realize that mothers do far better, before and after delivery, when they realize that medical concern embraces the entire family unit. My own hospital, Beth Israel in Boston, has recently adopted a family-centered maternity care program. Its goals are to insure that the mother has the best possible experience during pregnancy, labor and post-delivery stay, enabling her to share this experience with the baby's father, both leaving the hospital confident in their ability to care for the baby.

The program treats childbearing as a normal healthy process, and as a major family experience for all concerned. Fathers are encouraged to be with their wives during labor and delivery, and are allowed to visit at almost any time during the day and evening. This is far more civilized and healthful than treating the men as invaders who must be herded into a waiting room to pace aimlessly or hold inverted magazines in their laps.

The husband is always important, and is welcome at the second visit. But don't be bitterly disappointed if he does not choose to come, for his reasons are valid, though probably unfathomable to a woman. Some men simply cannot think of themselves sitting in a waiting room in the presence of several pregnant women. It's not so much male vanity as it is inhibited composure. This may not make much sense to wives, but then, neither does a groom's need for a stag night.

If your husband does choose to accompany you, the doctor will very quickly put him at ease and point out how helpful he can be during the coming months—especially with such necessary disciplines as weight control, diet supplements and exercise.

But if he is not there, make it a special point later to brief him on everything that happens. He wants to participate in this project whether he can admit it or not, so he'll be glad to receive a full report.

Routine for all visits is a urine specimen, so another will be taken. It will be tested for the presence of sugar and albumin. These tests relate both to possible problems of the pregnancy itself and to physical problems in the woman that might affect the pregnancy. Blood pressure is also checked at each visit, because changes beyond those normal to pregnancy alert the doctor to any limitations in heart function and blood flow.

The doctor will also appraise the physical changes that have taken place since his first examination. The most obvious is in weight, probably a gain. Since the birth package is still quite small, most of the added weight must be assumed to be yours. This ratio is scheduled to change each month until, during the last weeks, nearly all of the gain will be the baby's.

Bodily changes during pregnancy are quite radical, which is why it is so important to monitor them each month. Special changes may indicate special procedures which are invariably more effective when taken early. Kidney difficulty and cardiovascular problems can also be dealt with more effectively through early detection.

Except in unusual circumstances you will probably not have another pelvic examination at this visit, or at any over the next several months. The doctor can learn what he wants to know simply by feeling your abdomen.

Patients are often amazed and sometimes skeptical to find that the doctor can get an accurate idea of the size of the uterus by feeling the abdominal wall with his hand. But he can, just as you can get an idea of the size of a ball by touching part of it. In a relatively thin woman, the enlarging uterus can now be nicely outlined low in the pelvic area, even though it is not yet big enough to be noticed in a casual glance.

An advantage of this brief examination is that it leaves plenty of time for questions. If your husband is present, he may have queries of his own on how he's supposed to live with a pregnant wife.

Don't be surprised at a certain degree of conspiracy between husband and doctor, as they agree to help you to keep your weight down, or to discourage you from severely arduous activity. The doctor is merely trying to make your husband an ally for the coming campaign.

Pregnancy causes a wide spectrum of moods and anxieties; both doctor and husband can help deal with them, especially when the doctor has an opportunity to describe the changes that might baffle the man who must live with them.

For example, a pregnant woman's energy output can be expected to vary surprisingly from day to day. Or she may seem buoyant with health at one time, then suddenly lapse into lassitude and moodiness. These shifts and switches are merely the signals that major changes are taking place within her body; if the husband understands this, he can make a few adjustments himself.

Particularly in the case of a man who likes a regular, predictable routine, it ought to be emphasized that pregnancy often finds normal rules offensive, and goes its own way. The husband who understands this can bend a little.

Around the time of the second visit there may be several discomfitures to report. Perhaps you've been having a backache that won't let up, or you're wondering why, instead of the simple fatigue you were led to expect, you got total exhaustion. Quite often women at this stage feel that they have become gross, inflated beings, despite the fact that weight gain is well within bounds.

These are all reasonable, typical complaints, not to be minimized simply because they are normal.

Anxiety is part of the picture, too, and no woman need hedge about it. A baby makes a monumental invasion of the body, and if it causes loss of emotional stability once in a while, allow for it.

A useful precept to cling to in the pinches is this: the major fact of pregnancy is change; no matter how you may feel today, you are not likely to feel that way tomorrow or next week.

The second visit to the doctor—with husband or without—can offer an opportunity for both partners to inform themselves of the specific methods by which the innocent invader can be expected to alter the pattern of their daily life.

Oddly, in spite of all these changes, many women at this stage are apt to insist, "But I just don't *feel* pregnant." The physical symptoms are distinct enough, but it is often hard for newcomers to relate them to the fact of a baby growing within them. At ten weeks or so the abdomen has not yet begun to bulge, there is no physical motion by the baby, and very little other tangible evidence is present to indicate meaningfully that a six-to-eight-pound human is actually under construction.

Therefore, if a woman finds this hard to believe, it is only reasonable that her husband may not accept it yet, either. Aside from noting that his wife may tend to smile a lot, it is often difficult for him to remember that she is not quite the same girl who was always ready for a night on the town or a walk on the beach.

But the changes are striking, many more are to come, and the husband must adjust to them as surely as his wife must soon start to adjust her clothes.

One of the most basic accommodations to be made is to a probable change in the woman's regard for sex. This is a matter of such importance that she should talk about it with her doctor and with her husband, together or singly, as candidly as possible.

A woman frequently becomes less receptive to sex during pregnancy, or at least less relaxed about it. If the pregnancy is unintentional or inconvenient, she may have less enthusiasm for the cause for a while.

There are plenty of women whose attitude toward love-making doesn't change at all, and quite often the fact of pregnancy seems to make certain women considerably more eager for it.

Whatever the case, self-examination of attitude is a good investment of time. Ideally, pregnancy should enhance a marriage rather than jeopardize it.

Ask yourself, is there any chance that you are unconsciously resentful about having been impregnated? Maybe you are needlessly fearful that love-making might injure the baby? Watch out also for the Madonna complex—the feeling that the experience of gestation is somehow too sacred to permit your husband's indulgence.

Once in a while, perhaps when trying to achieve a pregnancy has been a problem, a woman may feel freer and more abandoned about sex. She should certainly not berate herself for enjoying it. Everything we know about human nature suggests that a man and a woman who live together in deep affection are intended to make physical love.

Another serious hang-up among some expectant women is that they feel they are no longer desirable. Wrong, wrong wrong! If your husband says he finds you irresistible, he is probably not kidding—you *are!* Most often a pregnant woman is radiant with health, she no longer has any concern about contraception, and there is an added excitement in the knowledge of what past pleasure is about to produce.

Probably the only condition under which the doctor might advise restraint or abstinence in love-making would be the presence of such danger signals as staining or cramps. But even if diminished sex life happens to be necessary, a well-adjusted couple need only to resolve openly that they will make the most of the times when they can get together.

Every physician who deals with pregnancy has a wealth of experience from which to give counsel on the role of sex during this time. Don't let inhibitions or social niceties prevent you and your husband from taking advantage of this useful information.

After the husband has become acquainted with the doctor, or after his wife has briefed him on the details of her latest visit, he may wish to ask the doctor questions directly, or have his wife make certain inquiries at later visits. This is perfectly proper and desirable, for it creates better understanding and often helps the doctor to achieve better management of the case. The man usually remains calm in times of stress despite that TV cliche about fathers who go to pieces at delivery time.

A husband is quite likely to emerge from a visit to his wife's obstetrician as a sort of instant expert on maternity; so why not let him be useful?

A matter of some importance at the second visit is the result of the previously taken blood test: the Rh factor. This poses no problem whatever if you are Rh-positive, as are some 85 per cent of patients. If both partners happen to be Rh-negative, there is no need for concern.

The Rh factor only requires special consideration when the woman is negative and her husband is positive. As you now read the full Rh story, remember from the outset that the threat this incompatibility once presented has been brought under medical control. Once a menace that baffled scientists, the Rh phenomenon is now little more than an interesting story of conquest over a disease through research.

When a woman is Rh-negative and her husband is Rh-positive, their offspring is most often Rh-positive, too. This means that there is something present in her husband's blood which will probably be passed along to the baby but is alien to her own system.

Medicine does not yet know the function or purpose of the Rh factor. Until 1939 it was not even known to exist. Before then, doctors were mystified by babies who unaccountably died of what was then called dropsy.

Then the Rh factor was discovered.

For several years after Rh matching began, there continued to be cases of women whose first babies suffered severe anemia or died. The reason was that at some time the woman had inadvertently received Rh-positive blood which had caused her to develop antibodies. These, if transferred to her baby, caused its blood cell destruction.

Mistakes in blood and Rh matching nowadays are rare and hardly worth mentioning. Furthermore, modern tests can now determine how much of a threat the mother's antibodies pose to the child she is carrying.

It might seem that the mother's blood would inevitably be brought into constant contact with her baby's blood and the hostile ingredient in it. But this does not happen. The mother's blood nourishes the baby, but not by circulating through its system, as is commonly thought.

For there is a remarkable apparatus at work in the placenta. The mother's blood arrives there, laden with oxygen and nourishment for the growing child. The baby's blood arrives there, too, but the two systems do not mix. There is a protective barrier that separates one blood flow from the other, allowing only the desired nutritional exchange. To complicate the system further, the baby's unwanted materials—carbon dioxide and waste—are also taken up by the mother's blood without any intermixing of the two circulatory systems.

But this barrier is not altogether impenetrable. At the time of birth, or shortly before, microscopic breaks can occur, and some of the blood can exchange. As some of the baby's Rh-positive blood enters the mother's Rh-negative system, she will begin to develop antibodies. As expected, she will carry these antibodies with her in the same way she carries antibodies against measles or chicken pox.

But since this response only begins near the time of birth, the first baby is separated from her body and is in no danger, since the hostile antibodies have not had a chance to affect that baby.

With second and subsequent pregnancies, however, additional small exchanges might occur, causing the mother to develop a stronger and stronger reaction to the Rh factor. Now that we have a method for measuring the degree of such response, an Rh-negative woman's doctor will know beforehand if her child faces a serious threat at birth time.

Fortunately today even the threat can be prevented. When the doctor knows that an Rh difference is present, the woman can be treated following delivery with an injection of a special gamma globulin (Rhogam). This is selected material from the blood plasma of women with a very high level of anti-Rh. If given within 72 hours after delivery, it will prevent the woman from developing Rh antibodies that would threaten a future child. The material is safe, widely used, and virtually foolproof in preventing Rh difficulties.

Very rare these days are instances in which the Rh factor poses a grave threat to a child. In such cases the doctor may elect to take the baby two or three weeks early, thus minimizing more the possibility that the hostile atmosphere might cause Rh antibodies to enter the baby's system through breaks in the placental barrier.

If the child is affected by Rh disease at birth, two methods of treatment are available. Most often the baby is simply placed under an ultraviolet light which helps to eliminate the toxic materials produced by the breakdown of its blood. If the condition is critical, gradual total replacement with fresh Rh-negative blood is necessary.

Sometimes, when a serious Rh threat of infant death exists before the birth, an extreme form of treatment has been tried: to transfuse the baby while it is still in the uterus. This technique is still in the developing stages and is available only in large teaching centers.

Altogether, any woman who finds herself facing the problem of Rh incompatibility can take comfort from the fact that she is the beneficiary of one of the most astonishing accomplishments of medicine: the discovery of a disease, the isolation of its cause, and the perfection of preventive control methods, all within 30 years!

One additional note of recent investigative work: Rh-negative women who abort in early pregnancy either naturally or for therapeutic reasons should be protected by Rhogam, even though the RH type of the fetus is unknown. The patient runs some risk of developing Rh problems and should be offered the same protection as the one who delivers her baby.

There is another reassurance especially important to women who are carrying for the first time: they'd like to be positive that their babies will be normal and healthy when they are born.

It would be marvelous if a doctor could just put a stethoscope on your belly and say, "Of course it will!"

But we must be realistic. It happens that babies *are* born with problems. But the odds against it are enormous. Only three of every 100 children born in this country are less than perfect. If that figure reminds you of your penchant for bad luck, add this to it: more than half of all such defects are so minor as to be insignificant. There might be a little patch of color at the back of the neck; it will probably disappear shortly after birth. Sometimes there's a slight mismatch in foot development, but a good pediatrician will spot it and start correction immediately.

Most other physical defects can be dealt with so skillfully that they will never be a serious handicap to the child.

Remember also that the 97-out-of-100 figure for normal births comes from the *entire* population. This includes thousands of women who never see a doctor, yet who bear their children under conditions ranging from privation to destitution. Therefore, if you are a healthy, well-nourished woman under regular prenatal care, you have already cut down on those odds considerably.

Pregnant women tend to worry and brood, at times, over possibilities that may have little or no basis in fact. Let's look at some of the other threats, real and legendary, that perhaps seem to lurk over your baby:

Suppose you had a dental, chest or other X-ray picture taken after conception, but before the pregnancy was confirmed, could it have affected the fetus? The risk is negligible because such exposures are so brief. If any X-ray is necessary during later pregnancy, your abdomen will be protected by an apron containing a heavy metal which will block out the rays. The use of X-rays in medicine has become so sophisticated that birth accidents attributable to it are only an event of the past.

Neither is there now much danger from the use of general anesthesia on a pregnant woman. When such gases must be used, the anesthetist uses a mixture that is high in oxygen. This gives assurance that in the event of a momentary drop in the mother's blood pressure—perhaps at a critical moment in the formation of the child—there will still be enough oxygen available in the placenta to nourish the dividing cells.

I said earlier that advances of medicine come along so quickly that portions of this book had to be revised just before printing. This is one of them. For, at this writing, one of the most terrible threats of pregnancy may be on its way to oblivion. The disease known both as rubella and German measles is now under attack by a vaccine.

Rubella has caused terrible tragedy over the years. Babies can be affected physically, mentally, or both, if the mother gets the disease in the first three months of pregnancy—the earlier the infection, the more devastating the toll.

Most women are immune to rubella from having had it in childhood. For the minority who have not, there are two recent developments that will help cut down the odds of this disease.

First, there is a test to determine if a woman is immune to rubella; this is now a part of routine prenatal blood workup. If she is one of the few who has not had the disease, she must be advised to take special care to avoid it.

When a woman suspects that she has been exposed to rubella during the critical period, this test will tell the story.

The second advance is a vaccine against rubella. By immunizing all children with the vaccine, the chances of their infecting pregnant women can be cut down sharply. The early vaccines are effective, but not ideal. Further studies are necessary to find the vaccine that will forever wipe out this disease.

Until the vaccine has accomplished its benevolent work, a woman may still contract rubella during the critical days of early pregnancy. Let's say she discovers that she has been exposed to rubella. Perhaps one of her children's friends will announce unexpectedly, "My brother's home with German measles." Or she may learn too late that the little girl who had had lunch with the family on Tuesday came down with rubella on Thursday.

The natural reaction to these situations? Panic. "I've been exposed to German measles, Doctor. Isn't there some kind of a shot I can get to help?" She's probably referring to human immune gamma globulin which is often given to protect people who have been exposed to viral diseases.

But in pregnant women, this material will do no more than minimize her symptoms. Masking these signs and symptoms cannot prevent congenital damage to the fetus. So I would never give this material to a patient exposed to rubella during her first three months of pregnancy.

If her exposure to rubella *has* resulted in infection, it will show up in a test later. Unhappily, there is nothing we can do either at the time of exposure or upon verification of the disease to prevent or correct damage to the child.

A major decision must be made at this point. A doctor can guide and counsel, but it is the mother who must ultimately decide.

First, she must be advised on the reliability of the diagnosis and the significance of the dates involved. If she is young, and can apparently conceive again easily, she might more easily want to terminate the pregnancy by therapeutic abortion. In such a case, her religion may be a determining factor.

The law of the land as proclaimed in January 1973 by the Supreme Court in Roe v. Wade entitles her to termination if she so desires; in this case she may be afraid of the high potential for damage to the forming fetus. It would be hard to fault her for requesting abortion, especially if she is young and has a promising reproductive period of life ahead of her.

Why can't the vaccine be given to pregnant women themselves? Because the vaccine could also cause damage to the fetus, in spite of the fact that it has been made weaker than the ordinary German measles virus. During the present, early campaign with the vaccine, the policy must be that no woman who is pregnant, or who might become pregnant in the next three months, should receive it. As the prevalence of rubella is reduced by mass immunization of children, we can expect that this policy will be relaxed. If the vaccination program is successful—and there is no reason to believe that it won't be—then women may be routinely fortified with a German measles vaccine booster as adults. But because the disease wreaks its havoc so early in pregnancy, it will probably always be necessary to determine that a woman is not pregnant at the time the booster is given. Unfortunately, it can be statistically predicted that some women will have babies who are victims of rubella damage in spite of the advent of the vaccine. But every day, the odds will diminish.

This chapter has probably dealt with the possibility of abnormal birth far more than will your third office visit, unless you ask the doctor special questions about it. If you have any qualms whatever, don't hold them back. Ask the man who has the answers, then put such thoughts out of your mind; your baby is now past the basic formative stage and these fears can be set aside.

You are also at a point which makes the findings of the physical examination quite interesting. For example, although your body does not yet announce publicly that you are pregnant, the signs are now unmistakable, and the doctor will duly note them for you.

Your breasts have enlarged and become quite firm. If you feel that Nature was less than generous to you in that region, enjoy the temporary pulchritude while you may; for after delivery and lactation your breasts will return to their pre-pregnant size.

By now the nipples have darkened, and the areola around each contains many small pebbly rises. These are technically known as Montgomery's follicles, but "little bumps" is just as good.

You have probably noticed an increase in vaginal secretion. This is because the glands of the cervix, like all glands of the body, secrete more than usual during pregnancy. The body is "busier," like a machine that has had its speed slightly increased, because it has much more to do. If the vaginal secretion is irritating, the doctor may permit a gentle warm douche.

But don't use a bulb syringe—*ever.* Use a bag, and hold it low. Too much water pressure can be dangerous at any time, and surely is in pregnancy.

In addition to increased discharge there may also be present a bothersome yeast fungus called moniliasis. For this condition a vinegar douche and vaginal suppositories are safe up until the eighth month, when the doctor will tell you to stop.

There may also be a cheerless surprise by now—a rash on arms, chest or abdomen. This is an unsolicited decoration of pregnancy that thousands of other women didn't plan on, either. Treat it with a lotion or cream that the doctor can recommend.

Ironical, isn't it, that so many major events should occur in you, while your husband remains absolutely unscathed!

There is one matter you can let him handle exclusively, if you like: the business of the doctor's fee, if it hasn't yet been settled.

New and broadened insurance coverages have taken much of the chill out of fee discussions, but there are still a few aspects of the financial arrangements that many patients misunderstand.

Contrary to common attitudes, it is perfectly proper to be frank and candid in talking about the money involved in a doctor's services. This includes asking if you are expected to pay in advance, or as you go along, or if you will be billed following delivery. In equal candor, you may be asked some questions about your income, which usually means the doctor will adjust the fee to it.

Simple, direct questions about money are never out of order. Asking them can prevent an unnecessary strain on the patient-doctor relationship you are now trying to develop. This relationship is too important to you to be marred by a misunderstanding about fee and payment.

So ask.

Questions are your share of every office visit. If you have compiled a list over the intervening weeks, bring it along. Above all, if you feel any gnawing fear or concern, inquire about it. Your experience at childbearing, even if you have had several babies, is too limited for you to brand any qualm as ridiculous.

It is perfectly natural to experience fears while carrying a baby; the only one a doctor cannot abide is the fear of asking him about anything that bothers you.

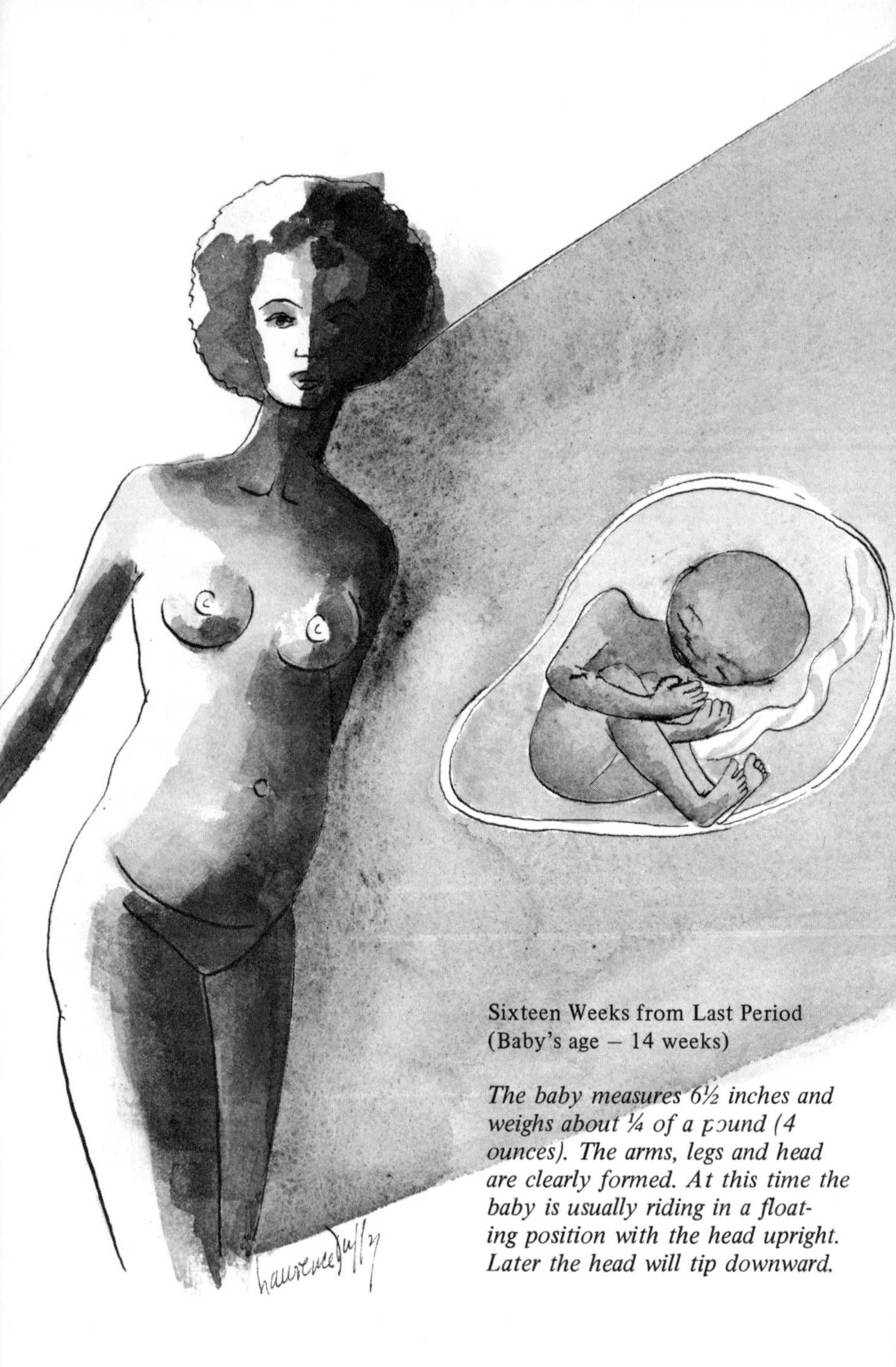

Sixteen Weeks from Last Period
(Baby's age — 14 weeks)

The baby measures 6½ inches and weighs about ¼ of a pound (4 ounces). The arms, legs and head are clearly formed. At this time the baby is usually riding in a floating position with the head upright. Later the head will tip downward.

THIRD OFFICE VISIT
IN THE FOURTH MONTH

the calorie battle is on!

Have you ever seen a doctor look askance? You will if your weight is high at Visit Number Three. The past 30 days have been a time of accelerated response to the fact of a rapidly growing baby within. This is the month in which many women seem to resign to their condition, excusing themselves for indulging the whims and wishes of appetite. They arrive for examination with much of this nourishment visible.

You were first weighed two months ago. If you carried extra pounds then, the doctor probably put great emphasis on the importance of holding down your food intake. Perhaps your weight was normal until you were beset with the ravenous appetite that pregnancy often unleashes.

The second weigh-in may have shown you to be about the same, or only slightly heavier. But since then have you been packing away calories gustily, confident that you were only doing your duty toward the hungry being inside?

My dear, he's not all that hungry!

Hearken again to the inflexible catechism of maternity: At term, the baby, the placenta, the bag of waters, the enlarged breasts and any weight gain of the body, including fluid, should not exceed twenty to twenty-five pounds altogether. Try toting this amount around in your hands for a few minutes and you'll understand the strain inherent in pregnancy. This is why pregnant women often feel soreness in their hips, knees and ankles, why they tire so easily, and why they feel out of balance much of the time.

For nearly all women, the process of gestation seems to demand more fuel than they would normally eat. They know they are expected to gain as the birth package enlarges, and they can't fathom where this extra material is going to come from unless they take it on in the form of extra food. The fact is, however, that the internal biological system can manage distribution much better than the eater can. If a woman were to fast during pregnancy, which, of course, she should not, her body would still know how to budget the materials on hand to supply what is needed for the baby. In spite of recent attitude changes on this dictum, most obstetricians still believe that weight control—so long as it does not deny necessary nutrients to mother or child—is worth its cost in self-discipline.

Perhaps it will help you to deal with the tendency to overeat if you understand why it is so important to hold your gain to the prescribed range:

A growing baby causes acceleration of all bodily functions. Each of the separate systems works at an elevated rate, and overtime, too. To saddle this response with the additional burden of useless weight is to lessen body efficiency.

An immediate problem is clumsiness. As the baby grows, the mother's center of balance begins to shift, so she is likely to move awkwardly anyway. She'll tend to lag a little behind in adjusting to the posture changes required by the expanding weight. If she also adds unneeded weight to her body, she heads toward becoming a gross, slow-moving thing, all stumbles and grunts.

From the point of view of vanity alone, a woman should realize that people can tell at a glance what kind of pregnancy she is engaged in. She can be neat, visibly healthy and aglow with anticipation. Such a condition makes her attractive—even sexy.

Or she can plod through pregnancy, fat and slothlike, as though producing a baby is more a disease than a pleasure.

For health, safety, comfort and appearance, it makes sense to deny the addition of every unnecessary gram over the minimum.

If you are unlucky enough to begin your pregnancy with excess lard, your problem is complicated. For it is unwise to attempt loss while the baby is developing. The best you can do is to make sure your pregnancy diet contains the nutrients needed by you and your baby, and that your weight increase follows the pattern of a normal pregnancy: 1½ to 3 pounds in the first trimester, and no more than 8/10 of a pound per week during the remainder.

If you have become pregnant after having fought the battle of the bulge nobly and long, you may reasonably ask the doctor for special help during this early period; for it does seem as though your body is conspiring against you, stimulating the desire to get as many goodies into your stomach as you can. Sheer will power and noble intent are just not enough.

Falter not—help is available. There are pills that help you to feel less like a starving bear, yet do no harm to your baby. You and your will power must do the rest. You must truly want to stay within the limit.

And don't bother inventing excuses to tell the doctor—he's heard them all. I've listened to women blame their January, February and March gain on a big Christmas dinner! Then it's the Easter ham that's responsible.

Or they'll insist they'd be all right if it weren't for those powerful cravings. Funny thing about the cravings of overweight pregnant women: everything they crave has a high calorie count. A craving may be only a yen to help make you *feel* pregnant. Crave harder to feel *slim*.

Why should you get so hungry if you were not intended to eat more? Fair question. This may result from the fact that the state of pregnancy lowers the amount of acid by which your stomach digests food, and this chemical change has a strange effect on your appetite. Not much research has been done on finding the reasons for the weird alteration in food desires that go with being pregnant. It may be helpful to accept the hunger as out of proportion and cope with it consciously. Who is smarter, you or your stomach?

A prime reason for so much emphasis on weight control is toxemia of pregnancy, a threat of the last trimester in which the body fails to dispose of harmful substances, ultimately causing severe distress to the mother and seriously endangering the baby. However, it is the pattern of weight increase rather than the actual poundage that indicates to the doctor a threat of toxemia later.

In nearly every instance where toxemia occurs, it can be shown that the mother gained excess weight. This is why routine prenatal care is so crucial to a successful pregnancy.

As for yourself, madam, obesity strains the heart. Pregnancy taxes your heart anyway, because there is an addition in blood volume of about 30 per cent. This is mostly a fluid increase, however, for there is not a proportional increase in the number of red cells available to carry oxygen. That means the heart must pump a considerably larger volume of blood to accomplish the same results. Any pregnant woman has a relative anemia compared to her normal, nonpregnant blood count.

Fortunately, the heart is built to take up this extra load. It beats a little faster and each of its thrusts is a bit stronger. But the margin of endurance is narrower.

If a pregnant woman takes on more weight than necessary, she begins to borrow on this narrowed margin. Excess fat and fluids make it harder for her heart to push the blood through her vessels, and the added resistance produces higher blood pressure.

Obviously, if a woman has a previously damaged heart, say from childhood rheumatic fever, excess weight very soon begins to signal real danger. In a diabetic woman especially, weight control is of critical concern all the way.

Complicating the weight consideration is the fact that calories are only one of the enemies. The other is fluid. Among the most radical changes in a woman's physiology during the process of carrying a baby is the balance between fluids and tissue in her body. The fluid level goes up rather sharply.

A certain degree of fluid retention is normal. But all pregnant women must be watched closely to prevent retention from becoming severe.

Fluid has weight—a pint per pound—and the bathroom scale won't indicate whether excess poundage is caused by fluid or calories. Furthermore, fluid can cause the heart as much extra work as can fat.

The combination of excess weight, fluid retention and elevated blood pressure can almost always be seen in women who later develop toxemia. We cannot say they cause the condition, for medical science does not yet understand the relationship. But we do know this: if you do your part in the management of calories, the doctor can help you with the problem of retained fluids.

Maybe you remember reading somewhere that the fluid of the body has just about the same composition as the water of the sea. The key ingredient is sodium chloride—common salt. None of us could survive without salt; ironically it is salt that is a mystery during pregnancy.

An abundance of it is already present in pregnancy because of the copious secretion of the hormone estrogen. From the moment of conception, an ever-increasing amount of estrogen enters the system, and its function is to support the pregnancy. In fact, most of the estrogen of pregnancy is produced by the placenta. Unfortunately, one of the side effects of estrogen is the retention of sodium, obtained mostly from salt taken in with food. It is probably this high level of sodium that causes the body to retain more fluid.

In some women, the fluid level is so sharply altered by pregnancy that it may become necessary to hold down salt intake. But food without salt is generally uninteresting. Many of my patients tell me that this restriction can be pretty tough to live with.

There are several salt substitutes on the market, but having tried them all, I can tell you they're no substitute!

One of the best ways to make saltless food taste better is to sprinkle it with fresh lemon juice. Real zest can be given to beef, chicken, lamb or any meat just by squeezing a crescent of lemon over it. It's amazing how people who insist they could not eat a serving of fried or broiled fish without its traditional dash of lemon have never thought of using the same trick on meats, salads and vegetables. Try it.

Salt is the culprit in fluid retention. In the build-up of solid weight, a major enemy is sugar. This means starches, too, such as bread, potatoes, rice, spaghetti and pastry. If you recall early biology, you'll remember that starch is changed to sugar in the mouth by the saliva, which contains an enzyme for that express purpose. The enzyme sends the starches into the stomach as sugars, which later appear on your body as the penalty for indulging in high calorie intake.

Sugars and starches, because of their prevalence in most diets, can be blamed for more fat than fat itself. But in some patients, diabetics in particular, they have an effect beyond the problem of weight. Diabetes, in a pregnant woman, requires such careful attention that most obstetricians will seek the assistance of a specialist to work with them throughout the pregnancy.

It is not necessarily disastrous for a diabetic woman to become pregnant; but because of the sensitivity of the condition, she must be treated as a diabetic first and a pregnant woman second. A diabetic woman can bear children, but the diabetic specialist is vital to the process. He will examine the patient as often as the obstetrician, usually at the two-week intervals between the obstetrical visits.

In severe cases, the patient might be seen by one or both of her doctors every week. When the two physicians consult closely, they can help keep a diabetic woman under good control so that she has a far better chance of going on to a successful delivery.

This extra medical attention need not frighten a woman who is diabetic; her team of doctors is merely trying to hold her to the middle of the road so that the nature of the disease will affect the pregnancy as little as possible.

The same is true of a woman who must go through pregnancy despite a damaged heart. It is true that the heart must carry a significantly larger load during pregnancy, but damaged hearts can do it. With the help of a doctor who has special knowledge of cardiac disease, a woman with a troubled heart can take advantage of techniques and medicines that enable her to complete the pregnancy without further damage.

If major problems offer so much promise of solution, how can minor ones be so annoying? Case for consideration at this visit: waste disposal. Why should bowel function be thrown out of kilter so frequently after conception?

The most common complaint is constipation. In addition to its discomforts, this condition brings on an attendant complication called hemorrhoids. These are painful swellings of the large blood vessels surrounding the rectum. Constipation is frequent among pregnant women, but hemorrhoids are just about universal.

Some control over these aggravations can be exercised by eating plenty of leafy vegetables and roughage. These foods provide bulk and also offer the compensation that they are quite low in calories. It may become necessary for the doctor to advise mineral oil or milk of magnesia, but a patient can count on less trouble from constipation and hemorrhoids if she can manage to down the vegetables and bulk foods that lead to regularity. There is a new concept that bran in the diet aids in easing constipation. It also has been shown to be an aid in the prevention of cancer of the gastro-intestinal tract.

This erratic phase of the digestive process takes us right back to weight again. By this time the gain should be about four pounds. The monthly increase from now to delivery should be roughly three pounds. The schedule is not inflexible, of course, but it makes a dependable, if arduous, budget to follow.

The bathroom scale ought to be part of an expectant woman's daily life. Get on it once each day, and at about the same time, under the same conditions. A good time is in the morning, after you have voided, but before you have eaten. Night clothes don't vary much in weight, but if you're a stickler for accuracy, remember that nudity weighs nothing.

Here's another incentive that may help psychologically in holding weight down: how are you going to look following delivery? Wouldn't it be wonderful if you could finish this whole business at the same weight that you were before you conceived?

It can be done. Be faithful in abstaining from the Fattening Four: bread, butter, potatoes and dessert.

And don't reward yourself with candy.

Obesity can easily sneak up on you, but pregnancy offers a positive sign of warning. Take a look at your abdomen, where the baby is just now beginning to bulge. If you can see a clean line of demarcation between yourself and your bulge, then you can be quite sure that the weight you have added is confined to the weight of the pregnancy itself. But if the line is indistinct, it tends to verify the figures you have been reading from the bathroom scale each day.

If it has been discovered from the first blood test that a woman is Rh-negative, the doctor must know the blood type of her partner. If he happens to be positive, now is the time, in this third visit, to determine whether she has Rh antibodies present.

The likelihood is that she has not. But if she has, the doctor will evaluate the significance of the potential danger and make plans for his management of the Rh problem. In the ever-diminishing number of cases where Rh antibodies are present, the doctor makes a note to make further checks, beginning at the seventh month or so.

A delicate note ought to be included here: If both wife and husband are Rh-negative, there can be no danger of Rh antibodies in the woman. But suppose the conception were to be attributable, not to the husband, but to a different partner—one who is Rh-positive? Then the possibility of Rh complication would be very much present, wouldn't it?

We like to assume sweetness and light, love and fidelity. But such is not always the case. For the Rh-negative woman, there is this special peril in a liaison outside of her marriage. It is mentioned here only as a remote possibility. But it is certainly one which any such woman must take into account and reveal to her doctor. Otherwise he will have no reason to give her the Rhogam protection she needs for any future Rh-positive baby.

By the time of the third visit many of the discomforts of early pregnancy are probably over. If the tendency toward nausea has not cleared up, the doctor will probably take vigorous action to determine whether the cause is mostly psychological, or whether unusually altered body function is to blame. Once in a while this nausea can be so persistent that the victim must be hospitalized for a time to bring the condition under control.

Early pregnancy nausea, like increased appetite, may be linked to the decrease in free hydrochloric acid in the stomach. This same shortage often produces heartburn and an uncomfortable, gassy feeling. The reason is that, with less acid present, food is not processed at the usual pace. It is an irony of the gestation process that while most bodily secretions are speeded up, acid flow in the stomach slows down, resulting in the series of discomforts that often characterize early pregnancy.

But this acid condition usually corrects itself. In cases where the nausea persists, and where no physical cause can be found, it must be assumed that emotional attitude is involved.

For there are women who unconsciously resent or regret the fact of being pregnant. They may suppress the emotion, but they can't suppress their guilt over such a feeling, so they may punish themselves by prolonged nausea. Others may suffer continued sickness because of disturbed home routine or alarm over the coming delivery. The situation becomes irrational because it is unconscious, and so cannot be dealt with by the reasoning mind.

When emotion and unfelt attitude seem to be interfering with the pregnancy, they must be dealt with realistically. Often this can be done best by the woman herself; she acknowledges that there is something which she won't admit to herself, and she searches for it. This mental process may be enough to correct the condition. A frank discussion with her doctor about the possible hidden causes is also helpful.

By contrast, the mental attitude of most pregnant women is one of happiness. They are happy about everything—happy that they conceived, happy to be a bit dizzy now and then, happy to see the start of a bulge. I suspect that a poll of obstetricians on why they chose that branch of medicine would reveal it was because it's such fun to be among women who are so constantly delighted.

Some women are even fascinated by the radical alterations they are going through. Although if you could show a young woman a picture of what she will look like in her ninth month, she might be scared witless, as she goes from day to day through pregnancy, her most common response to the surprises is delight.

Stretch marks on the abdomen are an example. These are called striae, and can sometimes be quite vivid. Yet they seldom really disturb the wearer.

Striae are longitudinal streaks that seem to be just under the top layer of skin; they continue to increase in size up to delivery time, the way a design on a toy balloon does as it is inflated. Following delivery they will fade, but will not disappear altogether. Sort of a badge of honor.

Sometimes the skin rash, mentioned earlier, persists beyond the third month. If so, there are several possibilities: too much weight has been gained, so that parts of the body are rubbing against each other; or the heavier period of the pregnancy occurs in summer, when more perspiration is present. Once in a while the rash persists when neither weight nor climate is a factor. The best that medicine has been able to do in this instance is to give the condition a fancy Latin name—*dermatitis gestationis*— and treat it with lotions.

(Sorry about that.)

If unusual vaginal secretion has continued, the doctor can very quickly determine if it means difficulty, which is seldom. Most often the best answer is one which I call the "magic pitcher treatment." Make up a solution of warm, soap-sudsy water, sit on the john with legs spread, and gently pour the mixture over the outer parts. The treatment is comforting, sanitary and effective.

At three months, labor and delivery seem a long time away, which they are. But there is one phase of planning that it is wise to take care of early: arranging for some kind of human help to have in the house during the first week or so after you bring the baby home.

Most women in this country can't afford trained professional help. But there are young girls willing to work for modest payments, and there may be friends who will be pleased to offer a hand. The point is that assistance with a new baby is important enough to arrange for however you can and as soon as you can.

To come home with a new baby and enter the maelstrom of full household activity may be too much. If help has not already been arranged for, you'll probably be far too busy then to go out and find it.

The ideal helper is one who will take over many of the jobs that relate to the home and few that involve the baby. This should be the mother's time to get acquainted with her child, especially if it's her first. Even if the helper happens to be professionally trained in infant care, she ought to be as much instructor as assistant, helping the mother to learn the joyful chores, such as bathing and feeding, but taking to herself those things that are tiring.

Mothers and mothers-in-law may *seem* ideal for such help, but frequently they are not. Tensions run high in the presence of a new baby, and can become explosive between conflicting personalities.

Late night feedings particularly sap a new mother's strength. The interruptions are just enough to ruin a night's sleep. If she is breast feeding she will still appreciate the assistance of someone who will change the baby and bring it to her. Her husband will often try to be helpful, and this, or the two A.M. bottle feeding, is one task he could take on.

The baby who will one day cause this commotion continues to grow impressively. It has entered the period of its lifetime when the most prodigious growth will occur; it must expand its present size more than a hundred times before birth. From now on growth will be mostly in terms of enlargement rather than formation, for all of the baby's organs and tissues are fully formed and developing independently but in balance with one another.

The mother's abdomen is noticeably larger, her breasts have become firmer and fuller, and her center of balance has shifted. Shortly, if not already, her clothing must make its first major concessions to maternity. This is the time in pregnancy when tapping the amniotic fluid (amniocentesis) can be done to determine if there are genetic problems with the fetus. This is especially important for women over 35. I'll grant you that 35 is an arbitrary age limit, but we do know that it is after that age that genetic problems such as Down's Syndrom (mongolism) are most prevalent. Not common — just statistically more evident. Why do we wait until this stage in pregnancy to perform the test? Well, we must wait until the bag of waters is large enough so we can "tap" it and get the necessary fluid to be cultured and grown in a genetic laboratory. It takes from 3 to 4 weeks for the cells to be evaluated and genetic problems identified if present. A negative tap does not eliminate the possibility of an abnormal child, but it will rule out genetic abnormalities. As stated above, it takes about a month to get a result, and this leaves just enough time to perform a 2nd-trimester abortion if the results reveal that the child will be born with a genetically disabling and untreatable deformity. Abortion, of course, may be done only if requested. There is no law that says that the parents *must* have the blighted pregnancy ended, but there *is* a law which says they *may*.

Amniocentesis is not without its risk — infection, bleeding, damage to the fetus, or premature labor. But if it is performed under proper auspices and with the use of sonography to locate the position of the bag of waters and the fetus, it can be done with a minimum of risk.

The procedure so far will provide guidelines to the parents as to a course of action with regard to the pregnancy. But the time is approaching when amniocentesis will be used to determine whether a fetus is lacking in certain nutriments which can be supplemented during the prenatal course. In this way the method will save pregnancies that otherwise might be aborted. A bonus piece of information can already be gleaned from amniocentesis by examining chromosome formation to determine the gender of the fetus.

If you don't mind the mystery being taken out of the remainder of the wait for delivery, you can at least eliminate half of the given name possibilities that are still under consideration.

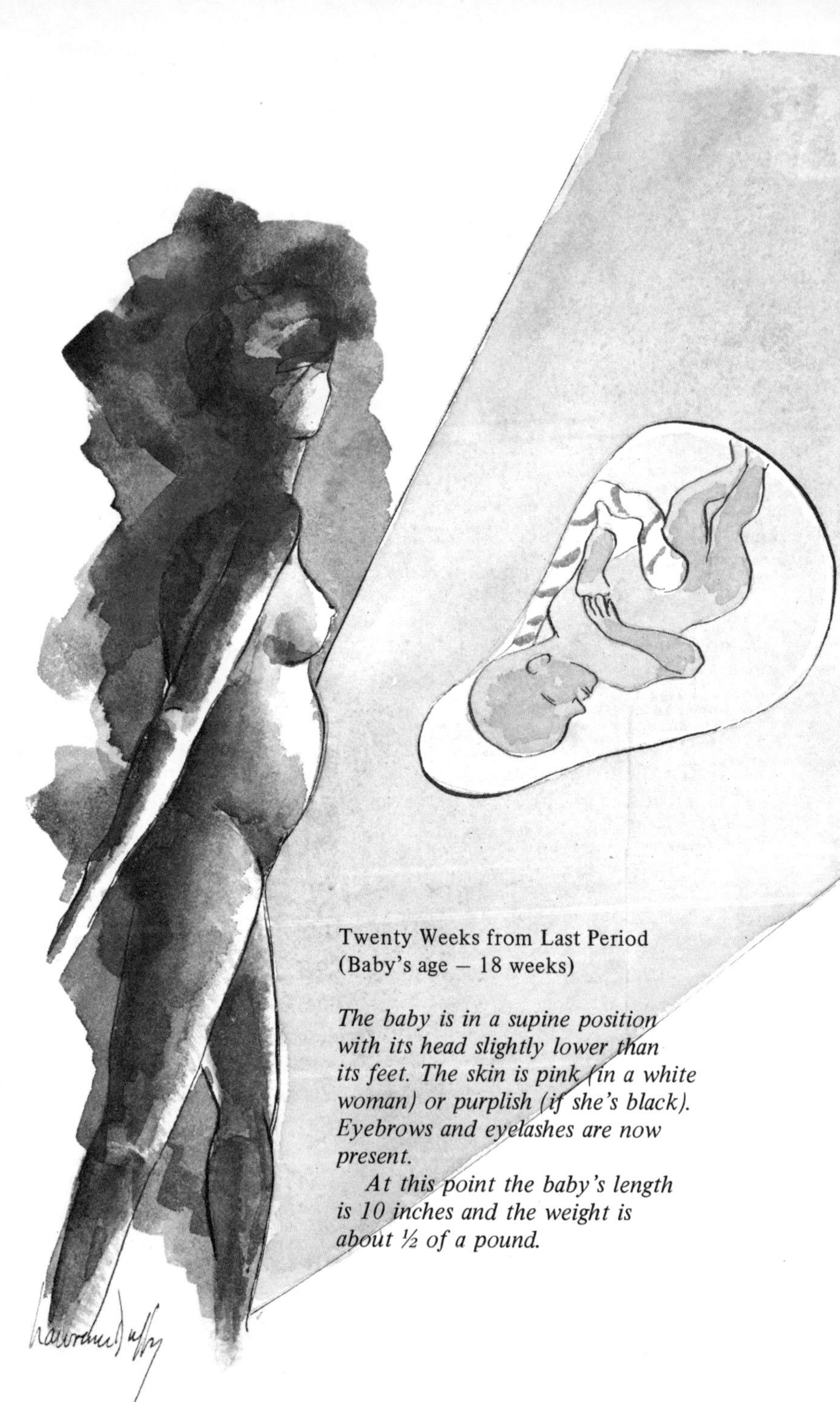

Twenty Weeks from Last Period
(Baby's age — 18 weeks)

*The baby is in a supine position
with its head slightly lower than
its feet. The skin is pink (in a white
woman) or purplish (if she's black).
Eyebrows and eyelashes are now
present.*

*At this point the baby's length
is 10 inches and the weight is
about ½ of a pound.*

FOURTH OFFICE VISIT
IN THE FIFTH MONTH

get the message yet?

One of the most exciting experiences of any pregnancy, but most especially a first, is that moment when the mother feels the first positive indication that she houses a living creature:

Her baby moves.

One of the great ironies of pregnancy is that women will wait eagerly for five months for the baby to move; then, when it does, they miss it.

There is no way, of course, that a man can describe the nature of this sensation, or its meaning to the woman who feels it. Some women say that the motion is subtle, some find it to be abrupt. Beyond that generality, medicine doesn't contain much of a guide as to how to describe the event to a woman who hasn't yet felt it.

(I must make a note to talk to a woman obstetrician who is also a mother.)

There's an important medical consideration that should be emphasized, however: if internal motion is *not* felt by the 17th or 18th week, the patient ought not to worry about it. Motion will surely be felt soon, and the sensible woman will simply wait for it. Sometimes a woman makes the absence of motion literally a matter of life and death. It is not. In fact, very often women slowly come to the realization that a series of subtle sensations which they couldn't identify were actually the first, feeble stirrings they had so eagerly awaited.

I have listened to *hundreds* of enthusiastic descriptions of early fetal motion, and have reduced them to the following scientific summation:

"Blip!"

If you have already felt a blip in your abdomen and have passed it off as nothing more than an abdominal blip, you have my sympathies.

An example of how subtle and misleading prenatal motion can be came out of a New Year's baby story. A 47-year-old woman who had never had a baby was taken to the hospital without the slightest suspicion that she was pregnant. (I think she weighed about 210.) When told she was about to deliver a baby she said she thought that all the action she had felt was just indigestion!

Accept this as a matter of faith: Whether or not you have identified an odd internal sensation as fetal motion by the time of the fourth visit, you have a completely formed baby within you. Cell division has reached that point where all of the organs and tissues have integrated in function and location. From now until term the process is one of growth and expansion. Motion will occur when the baby finds it expedient.

This is the time when the doctor begins to listen for the fetal heartbeat. His stethoscope may find it, but perhaps not, for it is still a very faint sound that is surrounded by a veritable bedlam that can be heard from the abdomen. There are gurglings of internal fluid, soft thumping sounds from the action or motion of organs, and miscellaneous other internal noises that make an infant heartbeat elusive at best.

We have, however, an electronic device called a Doptone that can locate and amplify a fetal heartbeat as early as nine or ten weeks.

This causes a very exciting experience, for the mother herself can clearly hear the beat from the loudspeaker of the instrument. It is not unusual in my office for women in the waiting room to burst into modest applause when they hear a baby's amplified heartbeat from the adjoining examining room.

A new height in sentimentality may have been reached by one young woman who had been thrilled by her baby's amplified heartbeat. Shortly after the visit, she returned to my office with a portable tape recorder. She made a recording of her unborn child's heartbeat and sent it to her husband, who was serving in Vietnam. She told me later that he played it every night before going to sleep.

This story reflects the importance of the heartbeat to the people involved, which is why it is touched upon here a bit early. If it happens that your fourth office visit falls at a time too soon for the heartbeat to be detected, take assurance that it will be easy to find next month. Or get yourself a military surplus stethoscope and let your husband fool around with it at home.

There is excitement and joy when an unborn baby's heartbeat is found for the first time. We must consider the sadness that comes in those rare cases where it is lost, indicating that the baby may have died in the uterus. This can even occur to women with good prenatal care. Sometimes it just seems to happen with no clue to the cause.

Such a sad event is hardly ever noted until after the 20th week. The threat of such a loss is possible when there is difficulty in the management of toxemia, diabetes, or kidney disease. In those conditions at least, the woman is able to prepare herself for this possibility. What is more tragic is the rare case when the pregnancy seems to be going along nicely, and the baby unaccountably dies.

In most cases of fetal death it is medically wise to allow the woman to continue until labor begins. This can be a bad time—the thought of carrying a dead baby can become so depressing that the mother's mental health may deteriorate. If her state of mind is seriously disturbed, the decision may have to be made to free her of the burden by surgery. Or a physiological problem—loss of a blood ingredient needed for clotting—may require the doctor to operate. But if there is no blood deficiency present, and if the woman can bear up psychologically after the mishap, she is better off to wait until natural labor begins.

Her body will react during this period by gradually lessening the activities of pregnancy. She will probably lose a little weight, her breasts will soften and return to normal size, and other signs of maternity will diminish.

This sad possibility ought not to be brooded over by a woman waiting for confirmation of a fetal heartbeat. Nor is the mere absence of fetal kicking a reason for panic, because unborn babies have been known to go for two days or more without letting their mothers know they are there. If the doctor finds the fetal heartbeat, that's all the reassurance needed.

Very rarely the heartbeat may be present, but undetectable.

Modern equipment makes it possible to take an electrocardiogram of the baby's heart through an instrument applied to the wall of the mother's abdomen. But until such a final test confirms that an infant has died in the uterus, there are always better grounds for hope than for despair.

Because of the fact that the baby is well-formed by the time of the fourth visit, medical considerations are now more applicable to mother and child together than they were earlier, when it may have been necessary to defer medical action. Certain treatments for the mother that may have been hazardous to the formation process can now be done with the risk reduced or eliminated.

Non-emergency surgery, for example, might now be done to ease the woman's delivery. This includes removal of ovarian cysts that can sometimes grow large enough to limit the expansion of the uterus or block the path of delivery.

Not only is the child fully formed at 18 weeks or so, but by this time the placenta has fully taken over the hormonal support of the pregnancy. It is well implanted on the uterine wall, and miscarriage is a very remote possibility.

Altogether a woman is in very good condition for surgery or other medical treatment. Most doctors feel, therefore, that this is the time to go ahead with any operation that will improve the condition of mother and baby.

Emergency surgery, of course, leaves no choice. At any time in the first four months, if an appendix kicks up, or a gall bladder becomes infected, action is demanded. An anesthesia rich in oxygen is used to prevent a drop in blood pressure, and special care is given during postoperative recovery.

It's amazing how pregnant women so often come through these emergency operations without compromising the baby. Still it remains an axiom in medicine not to operate until after the fourth month unless absolutely necessary.

Any surgery performed in or around the birth canal prior to pregnancy usually means that a normal delivery may be ruled out. This includes previous operations on the bladder, the rectum, the cervix, the vagina and the uterus. Surgery in any of these tissues results in large amounts of scar tissue, some of which may break down and cause hemorrhage if normal labor and delivery are attempted.

Women who have had such surgery are usually told quite early that their babies will be taken by caesarian section, if that is the doctor's policy.

If it is not, the patient herself has a stake in the decision. She is not a physician, but she is the one who is exposed to the risk of hemorrhage. Therefore she has a perfect right to ask her doctor to satisfy her that normal labor and delivery can be attempted safely. Conversely, if the risk of scar breakdown appears to be slight, she has the right to decide whether to accept the risk of a normal birth as described by the doctor.

Obviously, decisions of this scope depend upon honesty and candor between patient and doctor. By now such a relationship should have developed between them. If it hasn't, there can be trouble.

There are certain matters which a woman may find it expedient to keep to herself. But if any of these have medical implications, her doctor must know about them. To avoid pussyfooting, I'm talking about a woman's sexual past, which she may try to conceal. If that past happens to involve a prior pregnancy or surgery near the birth canal, she *must* confide in her doctor. Most often he will discover it for himself anyway. The fact of a previous baby, even when the woman insists she's carrying her first, is pretty hard to conceal from a physician.

But suppose a woman has had a past medical experience that leaves little or no trace? The doctor can thus be ignorant of a condition that is crucial to his management of her delivery.

There is a vast difference between a woman who has never carried before and one who is going through it for a subsequent time. The field of obstetrics makes a formal distinction between the two by the use of the terms *primipara* for the first, and *multipara* for the others. The treatment of each during labor and delivery is so distinct that each patient is designated one or the other when she arrives on the maternity floor. A woman who tries to fool her doctor is therefore actually only fooling herself and risking the loss of her baby.

When the doctor knows the facts a woman has tried to conceal, he has a subtle way of communicating that knowledge to others in the hospital who must also know if they are to do their jobs correctly. The woman is designated as a "social" *primipara*. This term tactfully informs the staff to behave toward her as though birth is a new experience, but to treat her as they must treat a woman who has delivered before.

But suppose that first birth involved a complication that might recur? The doctor knows she delivered—she bears unmistakable scars that show it—but because she has been deceptive, he can't anticipate the attendant problem.

If a woman finds it necessary to conceal the fact of a prior baby from her present husband, her doctor is bound by ethics to mind his own business. But *he* must know the facts.

A comfortable way to inform the doctor is like this: "I'd like to tell you in confidence that this is not my first baby." Or, "I've had surgery and treatment that I want you to keep in confidence."

Doctors are not judges; they are servants to your body. When you tell your doctor what he needs to know to serve you well, it becomes his responsibility not to say or do anything that might reveal what is to you an important secret.

Though the bulge is local, the pregnancy is general; it can't be used as an excuse to neglect such things as dental care. Sound health is a major objective for the whole period, including teeth and gums that are free of trouble.

Just about the only effect that pregnancy will have on dental problems is that bleeding gums will bleed more. It happens to be a deplorable fact that most people don't know how to include their gums in their daily dental hygiene, so it is not at all surprising that gum problems tend to flare up during pregnancy. Carrying a child does not cause gum disease, but it can often be a time when a woman finds out that her own dental care has been inadequate.

If you have been told that your unborn baby is raiding your tooth structure to get calcium for its bones, don't believe it. The myth of "a tooth for every child" persists. But it is not true. Any pregnant woman who is eating sensibly is taking in enough calcium for herself, her baby and both sets of teeth.

Any competent dentist knows how to alter his treatment in deference to a working pregnancy. In the early months, he'll make certain that his patient is not sensitive to a local anesthetic that could produce a shock that might momentarily cut off the supply of oxygen to the fetus. If extensive extractions are necessary, or if there is work requiring large amounts of anesthesia, he will consult the obstetrician first. When oral surgery is necessary, it can be done in a hospital with an anesthetist assisting.

If a patient has heart complications, her doctor will want her well fortified with antibiotics for extensive dental surgery. The important consideration here is to guard against the possibility of an infection settling into an already damaged heart valve.

Infected teeth and gums cause plenty of distress all by themselves. The possibility of such infection invading the body is reason enough to regard dental problems as threats to the pregnancy and worthy of thorough treatment as they arise.

What about a woman's own care of her body in this period when it behaves so differently? She likes to be clean and dainty, but often she feels—or is told—that ordinary habits of hygiene are forbidden.

Cleanliness itself, of course, is never forbidden, though some doctors are concerned with the method. They believe there is the risk that sitting in a bath may permit the passage of contaminated water through the cervix, therefore they rule out tub bathing. Others impose this restriction only for the last month before delivery.

I believe there is no serious risk in taking baths. Many women find that soaking leisurely in a bath is one way they can get the rest and relaxation that are often so hard to come by in some phases of pregnancy, so I don't like to deny them this pleasure unless necessary, which is hardly ever.

But a woman should not take a bath if the bag of waters ruptures at home and she is allowed to remain there for some reason. Labor is quite certain to begin shortly after this break, so there isn't time to sit around in a tub anyway. If she feels that she must make herself clean before going to the hospital, she can take a shower, which is perfectly safe.

Some doctors also forbid the taking of baths immediately following delivery, but medical support for this dictum is hard to find. In fact, for the tenderness caused by episiotomy—that's the incision made to ease the passage of the baby—one of the most comforting treatments is a sitz bath in two or three inches of water. Patients report that this does wonders.

Since we now are able to achieve excellent prevention and control of infection, many of the old restrictions can be dropped.

During the coming weeks there is likely to be plenty of internal action from the baby, and it may be hard to get accustomed to. Women usually interpret these motions as kicking, which probably does account for most of it. The baby has considerable mobility at this state, so it may be an elbow that you feel gently jabbing, or a sudden motion of the head.

The best guess is feet and legs, however, for the baby is now probably in a supine position with its head slightly lower than its feet, which are closest to the front wall of the uterus.

Our society seems to have emerged from that era in which pregnant women wore yards and yards of extra cloth to conceal a fact which the yardage itself helped to advertise. Modern woman has gone so far as to demand blue jeans with built-in expansion flaps as her work clothes during pregnancy. Her dresses may make no pretense at trying to hide that which obviously can't be hidden anyway.

So don't look for detailed advice on maternity clothes from this source. Learning obstetrics was simple compared to trying to understand what a woman, pregnant or otherwise, thinks looks good on her.

The best a doctor can do is to advise a woman to avoid any style or mode of the moment that makes her or her passenger uncomfortable. High heels, for instance, which seem to come and go from one season to the next, don't make much sense for a woman whose center of balance changes a centimeter or two every day. She looks forever poised upon a ski slope while standing, and her first impulse on sitting down is to take the heels off because they are too tight for her swollen feet. I'm told that the term "sensible shoes" seems to suggest something between an army boot and a brogan, so it is probably pointless to advise them. But if you can find shoes for dress-up occasions that sacrifice a smidgin of style for a bonus of comfort, you'll probably have a happier time out.

There is a garment sold that is known as a maternity girdle. I can't imagine a less appropriate term; it had nothing to do with accomplishing maternity in the first place, and its purpose seems to be a futile attempt to inhibit the fact once accomplished.

Many women believe that wearing such a contrivance will insure a flat abdomen with good muscle tone. It won't. The belly is intended to expand during pregnancy, and the woman is intended to get it back into shape afterward through exercise. A maternity girdle can only inhibit the expansion while it's taking place and weaken the muscles that are intended to carry the load.

In some cases where women are plagued by low backache, a girdle or an orthopedic appliance may be helpful; but it must be carefully fitted so that its support is in the back, not up front where the passenger rides.

Girdles seem to have become something of a security symbol in recent years, so much so that many women don't feel properly dressed without one. If you feel vulnerable when ungirdled, then wear it, but at least be sure it does not become tight in front as you enlarge. Too often a patient who is not doing well with her weight control will try to minimize her failing with fabric. Some even weigh themselves with it on, then blame the gain on the weight of the girdle. Guess whom they fool!

A maternity bra is something else. The breasts do enlarge and become heavy; they deserve the comfort and support of a special garment. Very often a patient will wear her maternity bra to bed to avoid discomfort when turning over, or when sleeping in positions in which the breasts appreciate support.

By this time in the pregnancy the breasts will have enlarged to their fullest likely extent prior to delivery, so that constant changing of bra size will not be a problem.

But for any woman planning to breast feed her baby, now is the time to refer again to the important bit of homework—toughening the nipple area so it will be ready for the assaults of a hungry and determined infant.

The most common cause of failure in breast feeding, even in a woman with plenty of milk to give, is that the baby may make the mother's breasts so sore and tender that she simply can't take the punishment. By then it is impossible to condition the breasts because they must heal first while the baby must still be fed.

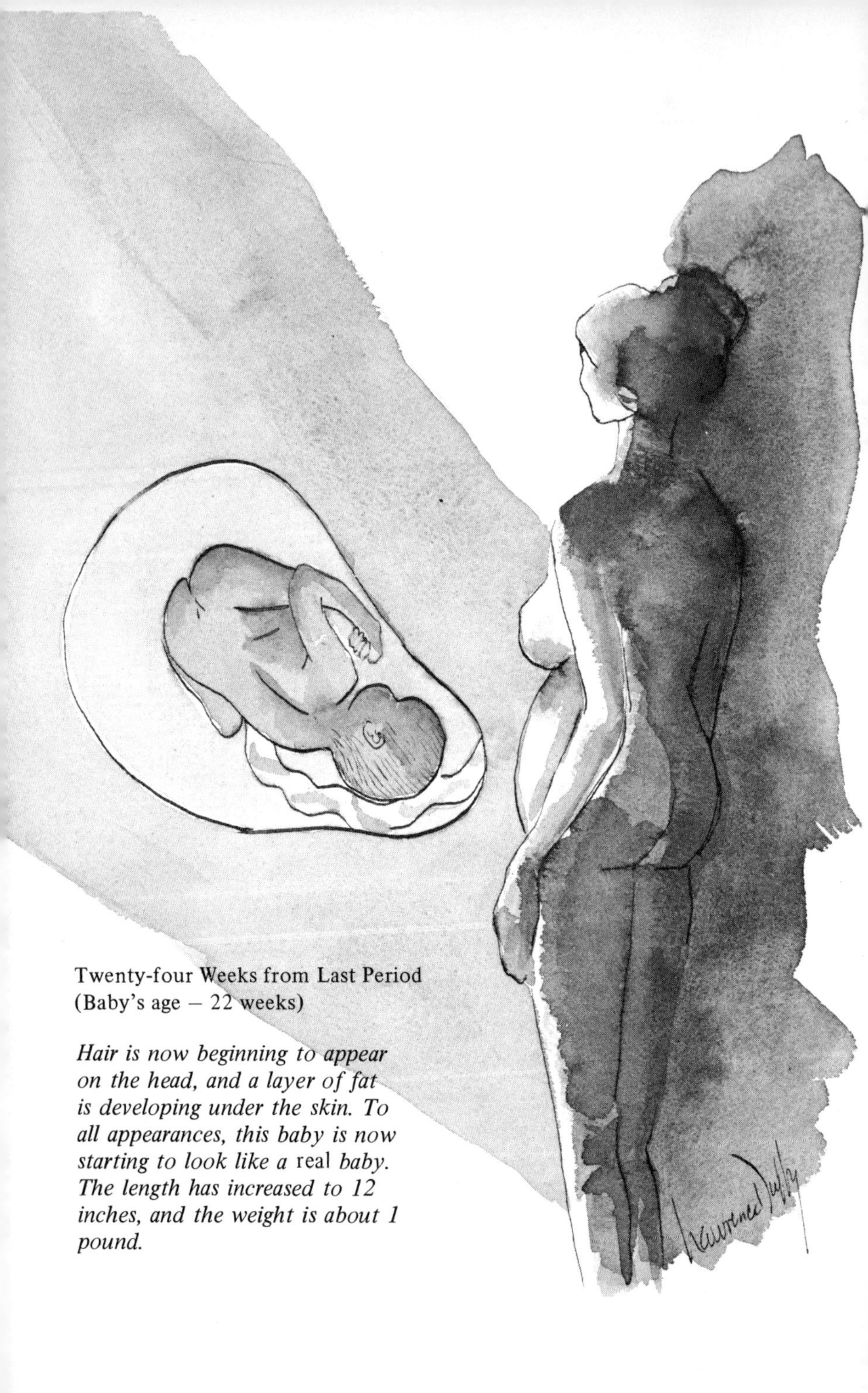

Twenty-four Weeks from Last Period
(Baby's age — 22 weeks)

Hair is now beginning to appear on the head, and a layer of fat is developing under the skin. To all appearances, this baby is now starting to look like a real baby. The length has increased to 12 inches, and the weight is about 1 pound.

FIFTH OFFICE VISIT
IN THE SIXTH MONTH

action on the home front

As the expectant woman contemplates the broadened expanse of her abdomen and realizes she still has about four months more to go, she has good reason to attach special significance to the old phrase "home stretch."

For all her girth, however, only about a pound, or 450 grams, is baby. During the remaining months that baby can be expected to grow to a weight of seven pounds or more. Further increase in the mother's weight, therefore, ought to be largely in terms of gain for the baby.

Perhaps the most exciting aspect of this fifth visit for the mother is that the baby's heartbeat is now unmistakable. This puts to rest the uneasiness caused by a disturbing occurrence she probably has noticed: For long periods of time there may be no detectable movement of the baby. Sometimes the interval is so long it becomes frightening.

But this happens simply because the baby, like every living organism, must have rest. Since an unborn baby has no consciousness as we know it, these rest periods cannot be called sleep. They are actually times during which the baby recoups its resources, just as the mother does when she goes to bed.

You probably have noticed that the baby becomes quite active when you are active. In moments of stress the fetal movements can be especially vigorous. This is probably because the baby's usual amount of oxigen is momentarily reduced, and his motions help achieve better distribution of the available supply.

It is also entirely possible that the internal fuss is very much like pounding on a radiator in a cold apartment to make the custodian send up more heat. A sharp kick from within is likely to make you gasp in surprise, and the gasp helps supply exactly what the baby is kicking for.

Next time you feel some unusual jostling, try inhaling several deep breaths. You'll probably notice that things will immediately quiet down.

When you are at rest, the supply of oxygen to the baby is usually regular and rich, so internal motion may be slight. If, however, you find that movements seem more pronounced while you are in bed, it is probably by comparison; you are not distracted by any action of your own, so you are more acutely aware of what the baby is doing. But vigorous fetal activity generally quiets down and seldom disturbs sleep.

Have you had the odd experience of suddenly feeling something move in such a way as to make your abdomen protrude? Now and then, in comparatively thin women, the sudden bulge can be touched and identified.

"I think it's a foot!" the woman will say in astonishment.

Chances are it is, indeed, a foot.

In examining you the doctor may choose to stimulate your baby into movement. He'll indent your abdomen with his fingertips, which causes the baby to squirm if it feels the pressure directly. But if the doctor's hand merely presses against the wall of the fluid-filled uterus, the baby will move away by displacement, pressing its body against the uterine wall somewhere else.

The baby is actually afloat, with a fair amount of free space for movement. The subtle motions felt are probably those of drifting, or shifting slightly within the chamber.

The space age gives us an excellent comparison for this condition: The baby is like an astronaut orbiting inside a space capsule. It is weightless in the amniotic fluid just as the astronaut is weightless in space. You are likely to feel its occasional soft contact with the uterine wall even without motion from its limbs.

The big thumps, of course, are made by the baby's legs, arms and head. Surely the origin of the expression "alive and kicking" could be traced to babies assaulting their carriers from within. In one way it is a comfort to know there's something doing down there, though sometimes the fracas can be more than a little distracting. If you haven't yet had a button kicked off, field-goal fashion, be ready for it.

This active tenant, at 22 weeks, has produced another set of changes to be noted by the doctor. The uterus has expanded, obviously, but it has also moved up out of the pelvis and is now located along a line just above the navel. The center of balance of the body from now on will be shifted only slightly as the birth package grows heavier.

If you have begun to have backaches from long periods of standing, it is most likely because you have adopted an inefficient posture to compensate for the new and localized weight.

If you stand tilted slightly backward, Tower-of-Pisa fashion, the weight will bear down so that it tires and cramps the muscles of the low back until they hurt.

This sort of backache almost never afflicts girls who are pregnant but not married. The reason is that in their attempts to conceal, or at least minimize, their socially unacceptable bulge, they pull in the abdomen and tilt the pelvis. Moral judgment altogether aside, this is an excellent way to carry a baby.

Posture alone, however, may not alleviate the back pains of pregnancy, because part of the cause must be blamed on the extra estrogen constantly produced by the placenta.

This hormone tends to relax the weight-bearing joints, especially those in the pelvis, lower back and hips. In the morning when a woman gets out of bed she is likely to feel loose, wobbly and out of balance, because these joints no longer fit snugly. The discomfort can be lessened by heat, massage with liniment, and rest. Here is a case where a maternity girdle *can* be of help. In severe pregnancy backache the doctor may arrange for othopedic strapping.

But proper posture accomplishes the most. Get into the habit of standing with your pelvis tilted slightly forward and your belly pulled in, and you will not only feel better, but you'll look far less like an impending disaster.

When you first began to expand, you noticed the stretch marks on your abdomen and the odd manner in which pigment was deposited in the skin to produce a pattern. Brunettes and black women who found rather pronounced stretch marks may now see a dark, well-defined line that runs downward from a point slightly above the navel. This is called the linea nigra, and is another result of irregular pigmentation as extra skin cells are grown by the body to allow for the necessary enlargement.

The same pigmentation may also now be more distinct around the nipples. Sometimes the areola—the circle in which the little bumps occur—becomes quite deep in color, matching the shade of the line down the abdomen. In blondes (if they are real) this area becomes pink.

I had occasion once to remark at a mixed gathering that the advertising slogan "only her hairdresser knows for sure" is far from accurate. For her obstetrician ought to be included. A blonde patient who was present gave me a look that could have broken Hoover Dam. What made it more embarrassing was that I had no idea, while she was staring me down, whether her blondness was real or chemical.

(Canon One in obstetrics: Learn to keep your mouth shut.)

Irregularity of pigmentation can also show up in a woman's face, making it something of a billboard of pregnancy. The effect is called "cloasma," the mask of pregnancy. There is nothing the doctor can do for it, but skill with cosmetics can help to hide it.

Sometimes women who are taking the contraceptive pill show the same facial coloration, though they are obviously not pregnant.

Very little scientific attention has been given to these colorations, probably because they usually disappear after delivery. One investigator has found that the distribution of iron is greater in the dark areas, but we don't know precisely how iron is related to skin coloring, or why it should change so noticeably during gestation. Whatever color a woman is, she is usually pretty much that color all over her body. Why some women become patchy when pregnant is not at all understood.

Suntanning will really emphasize the cloasma and darken it considerably. However, there are now creams and lotions called "sun screens" that will effectively block the sun from the affected areas.

There's a strange psychology among pregnant women: the more their bulge becomes visible, the more they think it is vulnerable. This is a logical conclusion, I suppose—if it's big enough to be exposed to knocks and bumps, there's a tendency to believe such assaults will be damaging.

But as was discussed earlier, a well-established pregnancy is rugged and durable. Miscarriages most often mean imperfect conception, not the fault of accident or trauma. A poor conception, indeed, may be shaken loose by an accident, but most obstetricians believe it was doomed anyway.

In spite of abundant evidence, hardly anybody believes us. If a conspicuously pregnant woman stumbles or gets bumped, those around her respond as though calamity had struck. The fact is that she is just as resilient when pregnant as she was when she was expected to jump up smiling after a fall on skis.

Yet the myth goes on. Any court case involving a pregnant woman becomes hopelessly lopsided because it is believed that the baby might have been hurt. Obstetricians get on the stand to testify that they find no causal relationship between an accident and whatever happened afterward to mother or baby, but judges and juries make big awards anyway.

For your own reassurance—if you choose to believe it—your baby is now wrapped in the safest, most efficient package ever devised. It can withstand fantastic punishment. I have seen a case in which a bullet passed through a woman's uterus without harming the baby. The wound was repaired and the pregnancy was not affected.

The traumas to your pregnancy also include children at home who are not above making a wild dash and a flying leap onto your portable mountain. As promised, they'll do no damage, but the act might be symptomatic of something that has happened to *them*.

Small children are unusually sensitive people. Though a mother may not have uttered a word about her condition, she shouldn't be surprised if they seem to know that something more is up than the unaccountable bulge.

Very often a small child will want to be picked up and cuddled more frequently. Some will whine, or sulk, or willfully raise local hell. This is just plain insecurity, based on changes in their mother that are felt but not understood.

Even when a child has been given no facts to go on, his intuition should be respected, and his mother should offer special comfort and assurance that he's not about to be relegated to an inferior status.

There is also a physical problem here; if the child is heavy and active, he can't be hoisted into his mother's arms as easily or as often. Give yourself a break; have the child hop up onto a chair before the hugging, or sit down and let him climb into your lap. Kids have more energy and less weight than you do, so they won't even notice that you are requiring them to supply the muscular output.

Love and attention are as important as food for children. Pregnancy is no time to start rationing either one. In addition to all of the other alterations of pregnancy, it must be a transition time toward a major change that will take place in the household when you come home with a new baby.

A sensible and practical approach to this transition is for you to combine your own need for additional periods of rest with your children's need for emotional comfort. Take a nap together, or just sit and visit, or play together.

As pregnancy becomes more tangible, you may want to begin introducing your child to the details he finds pertinent.

A small child can be absolutely fascinated by feeling for kicks and thumps from your abdomen. He can also be counted on to ask some of the wildest questions imaginable, because his mind is still uncontaminated by the inhibitions related to the sexual process.

I know a woman who tried to tell her child, gently and tenderly, about the baby that was growing within her, and how it sometimes made her tired and irritable because it was so heavy.

Unimpressed and unsympathetic, the little boy asked her, "Why don't you take it out and stick it in the freezer?"

At least she got a laugh, and so can you from these occasional sessions of relaxation with children who haven't the faintest idea that they went through the same process of production. Such visits are reassuring and educational, and blissfully restful for you.

It's a very nice arrangement.

Now let's see if I can muster as much enthusiasm for the idea of bringing small children to an obstetrician's office.

Sure, they'll be a problem, but they are entitled to at least one shot at it. Such a visit can be enormously important to them. They get to meet the doctor their mother has been talking about, and they are able to move one step closer toward acceptance of a situation that may be completely unbelievable to them. A baby is inside Mommy's body? Impossible!

A child can be totally hostile to the idea of your bringing home "a little brother or sister" for him. As Dr. Haim Ginnott has pointed out, this can strike him as no more acceptable than it would be to your husband if you announced, "I'm bringing another man into the house, so you'll have company."

A youngster who has had exclusive rights to his mother is especially disturbed by the changes in attention and routine that are caused by a new pregnancy. If he is interested at all in what's going on, it is in terms of how it's affecting *him.*

A common misunderstanding of mothers is that they think his target of resentment and jealousy is the unborn brother or sister. It is not. He's sore at *Mommy,* for all kinds of reasons: She's taking pills, she's weighing herself, she's making baby clothes, she's talking about the hospital. And she's telling him that someone he doesn't know and can't comprehend has become extremely important.

She has already begun to displace him, and he doesn't like it.

An obstetrician can only offer advice as to how these disturbances in other children may complicate the problems of pregnancy. For advice in handling the offended children, check with Drs. Spock and Ginnott.

Along about this time you may have a couple of other complaints that crop up in mid-term.

You're sitting in a chair, or lying in bed, when suddenly a muscle in your calf will seem to tie itself into a granny knot. These cramps come without warning and they hurt like fury. The most effective way to relieve the pain is to get some weight on the muscle in a hurry.

This is almost a reflex action, but it may need some training. At first you may leap out of bed with a shriek, scare everyone in the house, and knock a few breakable things over as you dance around in the dark.

There's not much to be done about such muscle cramps, either as prevention or cure. The knotted muscle can be kneaded and massaged, but the best initial treatment is to get it moving vigorously, in spite of the pain.

Cramps of this kind can strike the feet and the thighs, but most often they hit the calf muscles. They cause no damage and they indicate no abnormality, but this will be of small comfort at the time.

They hurt plenty! It was once thought that muscle cramps were caused by a low blood level of calcium, but boosting the intake of that mineral during pregnancy hasn't eliminated the occurrence of such spasms.

A heating pad will help to relieve the soreness after an attack. Or get your husband to massage the muscle for you—assuming, of course, that your shriek woke him up.

How are your ankles—sore and swollen? This discomfort relates to the change in fluid balance within your body that was described earlier. These symptoms can be found even though you are not gaining excessively and are keeping your fluid intake within bounds. After a long period of standing, the ankles can begin to hurt and shoes seem to be binding. You can get some relief by taking off your shoes and lying down with your feet elevated.

When fluid is badly out of balance there may also be swelling of the hands, making them look puffy, and enlarging them so much that a ring won't come off.

To remove a stuck ring, soak the hand for a few minutes in cold water, then, with the hand raised and pointed upward, soap both ring and finger. If you're sentimental about not wanting to remove the ring that was put there by your husband, park it on a knuckle until the swelling goes down.

Yet another bodily surprise is one at the scene of the action. This is a spasm, or contraction of the uterus. Sometimes it will start when your calendar says it's far too early for labor, so it obviously needs an explanation.

Actually, the uterus contracts regularly all during a woman's life, pregnant or not. The uterus is an organ equipped with smooth muscle—the kind whose actions are involuntary, like those of the heart and the stomach. A nonpregnant woman won't feel the contractions because they are too subtle. But they carry on with their rhythmic spasms as though rehearsing for their intended function.

From about mid-pregnancy on, when the uterus is enlarged, its contractions may become obvious. A small, hard lump will form in the center of the abdomen, hold itself poised there for a short interval, then disappear. A bit later, 15 minutes to half an hour, another such spasm occurs. It's a little bit eerie to find your body performing this way, but it must be accepted as another mysterious part of the reproductive process.

Later, near term, this normal activity can become a real problem for the woman and her doctor. Sometimes the contraction is accompanied by a twinge of pain, similar to a menstrual cramp. Has true labor begun, or are these just more intensive manifestations of the muscular tide to which the uterus is permanently committed?

A woman can help make the important distinction by careful observation of the exaggerated uterine action. If the abdominal lump can be dispelled by changing position, or by getting her body into motion, it is unlikely to be real labor. When measurement of the time interval between the episodes shows that the period does not become shorter, it is unlikely that real labor has begun.

Being pregnant can seem as though your mind has suddenly been transplanted into another body. Uterine contractions come as a total surprise. By the same token, you may find that although you have been ruggedly healthy all of your life, all at once you now have a tendency to faint. This can happen in any and all months of pregnancy. Most women do not have fainting episodes; but those who do can minimize the frequency of these spectacular and embarrassing events if they understand the cause.

Fainting is a most practical bodily mechanism. It happens when the brain does not receive enough oxygen, and so reacts by slowing down consciousness, or shutting it off completely. The result of a faint is that there is no longer the conscious control necessary to keep the body upright, so it falls over, thus lowering the head enough so that the blood needed can flow in without fighting the law of gravity.

Crude, but efficient. One way or the other, your brain is going to get the oxygen it needs.

Since falling down in a total faint is inconvenient, ostentatious and dangerous, you might as well seek the same result sensibly. When you feel faint, get your head down. Sit down, put your head as close to your knees as it will go. Put your hands on the back of your neck, push up with your head and pull downward with your hands. This will make your blood flow immediately to where it is most needed.

If you can't sit down or bend over, then lie down somewhere, floor or sidewalk not excluded. It may be awkward, but it's generally a better deal than a nose dive.

What you are doing is to help the parts of your body that are farthest from the pump. The heart is favoring its flow toward the baby, which is abetted both by gravity and proximity.

The same condition that causes faintness may also produce tingling in your hands and numbness in your feet. They, too, are far from the pump, and now and then will suffer from low priority.

Faintness most commonly occurs with abrupt motion—if you zoom up out of bed, for example, or if you jump out of a chair in which you've been relaxed for some time. Remember that pregnancy produces a larger volume of blood, but not an equally larger number of red cells to carry the necessary oxygen. Sudden bodily action calls for a sudden requirement of oxygen, but your thinned-out blood is not able to deliver it, so you get the flop-overs.

A woman who learns that she has a tendency toward faintness can exercise considerable control over it. She can anticipate the situations in which keel-over is likely. By moving slowly, and by taking deep inhalations of breath, she gives her body a chance to deliver the oxygen to her brain.

Probably the most acute situation for fainting is in standing up quickly after bending over. The blood in the brain spills downward, depleting the supply of oxygen to the cells of the body least able to withstand a shortage. They must tip you over, for that is the only way they can restore the flow without which they will perish.

The tendency toward faintness does not necessarily indicate that a woman is frail, or ailing, or that something is amiss in her pregnancy. She might be booming with health, yet she senses impending swan dives several times a day. This can only be blamed upon the change in the ratio of red blood cells to the total volume of blood fluid established during pregnancy, and we don't yet understand fully why it sometimes changes so radically.

The adaptability of a woman to labor and delivery is not necessarily proportional to her state of physical fitness. Most often a high athletic capability will be a distinct asset; a woman who is in good shape will do better than if her muscles are out of tone. A siege of illness, an accident, or a physical handicap obviously can be expected to reduce the body's capacity to labor and deliver efficiently.

But apart from these exceptions, it is difficult to predict how any woman is going to perform in labor. Among women in general, the thin, the fat, the frail and the rugged, there seems to be some sort of common denominator.

The body makes its demands, and somehow the demands are usually met. For labor is a great equalizer. There is no guarantee that a woman who has spent much of her life in spirited physical activity will automatically labor less or deliver sooner than one who has been waited on.

This is by way of preamble to the currently popular idea of a woman "preparing" her body for delivery by special exercises. Such a program of activity is required in the various methods of so-called "natural childbirth," or "prepared childbirth."

I quarrel with the terms because there is an implication in them that the doctor is to become a competitor rather than an ally. A woman in such training may be saying to herself, consciously or otherwise, that she is out to prove she doesn't need her doctor's help. This is fine, if she succeeds. But it is entirely possible for her to encounter problems that have nothing whatever to do with her own preparation, and which, therefore, do not brand her as a failure if her doctor ultimately determines that she ought to have help—medication, anesthesia or manipulation from him.

I have to be candid here. In 1962 I wrote a book that presented my reasons for opposing natural childbirth as it was practiced then. It seemed to me then—as it still does quite often—that many women were attempting natural childbirth for the wrong reasons and striving for the wrong results.

The training was aimed not so much at easing the pain of labor as it was toward proving how much the patient could take. We still see some of this pointless exhibitionism in the labor rooms. Sometimes it is even abetted by an insistent husband who is demanding a performance from his wife, just as he will later probably demand a performance from his son in Little League or his daughter in toe-dancing.

But there have been improvements, and I am happy to recognize them. Many sensible women now enter into prepared childbirth training determined to do the best they can, and thus to savor the rewards of the entire experience. They aren't out to prove how spartan they are or how little they need the doctor. They understand that delivery is an event of joy, not a contest. And at last the prepared childbirth husband is beginning to behave more like a sympathetic rooter and less like a demanding coach.

To prepared childbirth hopefuls I say this: I, like most other obstetricians, am delighted at your high intentions. But I hope my patients will take my word for it when I tell them they are up against problems that their rehearsals could not cover.

One out of every ten births will have complications. That is a fact; it makes no difference whether or not that tenth mother happens to be a disciple of natural childbirth.

What *is* accomplished by the exercises, whether for natural or assisted childbirth? They are commendable, of course. Anything done to improve the tone, coordination and power of the body is an addition to health and an expansion of capacity. But the exercises are not a preparation for miracles.

This is not intended to alarm any woman who happens to feel in marvelous health at 22 weeks. It is only to modify the unbridled enthusiasm with which many women sail into a birth-preparedness program as though its sole objective is to enable them to thumb their noses at their doctors.

Go to it! But don't expect that it will guarantee an effortless, painless delivery. For if this baby decides to aim itself the wrong way, or if it is headed toward a pelvis not quite big enough to permit easy passage, your record of rhythmic breathing and leg hoists will not change the situation.

Exercise classes often produce impressive results. They tone up the body physically and buoy up the spirit psychologically. So far as pain is concerned, we find that some women really do learn how to manage mind and body so that discomfort is minimal.

But for those for whom the method proves to be insufficient, there should be no qualms about accepting assistance and relief.

Preparation classes can have a very positive social value. Women facing the same experience get together to deal intelligently with the requirements. "Here we are, all in the same boat."

They learn more about their bodies and about the process taking place. They are also offered a constructive diversion from the less pleasant phases of pregnancy.

As for the exercises themselves, they are probably no better and no worse than any other program of bodily activities that expend the same number of calories over the same period of time.

A woman who plays tennis, rides a bicycle or takes long walks probably gives her body just as much specific conditioning as the one who specializes in calisthenics contrived to expedite the birth process alone. For fitness results from *usage*. Cycling improves the heart as much as it improves the legs that do the actual work. A good walk does as much to clear the brain as it does to take the kinks out of leg muscles.

Whether you choose to work out formally in a class designed for prenatal conditioning, or to exercise alone in an activity you enjoy, your reward will be in terms of time and energy invested, not of the particular muscles moved.

Any woman who has always been active and busy need not feel it absolutely necessary to prepare her body for the effort that lies ahead. But it will be a *maximum* effort, for which good conditioning will be an asset.

The subject of activity also includes consideration of whether a woman who holds a job should give it up because of her pregnancy. From a medical point of view, there are very few instances in which she must stop "for the sake of the baby." Not many women handle a rivet gun or carry the hod, and if more did, more would probably also do so while pregnant.

But there are many jobs where the presence of a conspicuously pregnant woman is unsettling to those around her; or where the work itself is not so joyful or rewarding as to make continuing it worth-while.

So far as pregnancy itself is involved, a woman can work right up to the time of labor if she chooses. The baby will ride out the activity nicely.

Speaking of His Prominence (or Hers), the obvious transition required here is, "Meanwhile, back at the paunch . . . ."

Very significant growth has taken place in the last month. The baby now measures about 12 inches in length. There is hair on its head and the skin is no longer transparent. At this stage the body is covered with a downy material called lanugo.

The weight of the baby is about a pound, which is very little for such a length. Though the baby is extremely thin, there is already a deposit of fatty tissue just under the skin.

A baby born at this time would struggle valiantly to breathe, but rarely could it sustain life for long, even with the help of an incubator.

Inside the protective environment of the uterus, however, this fragile child is lively and active. Never again in its lifetime can it match the rapidity of the growth process that is now going on.

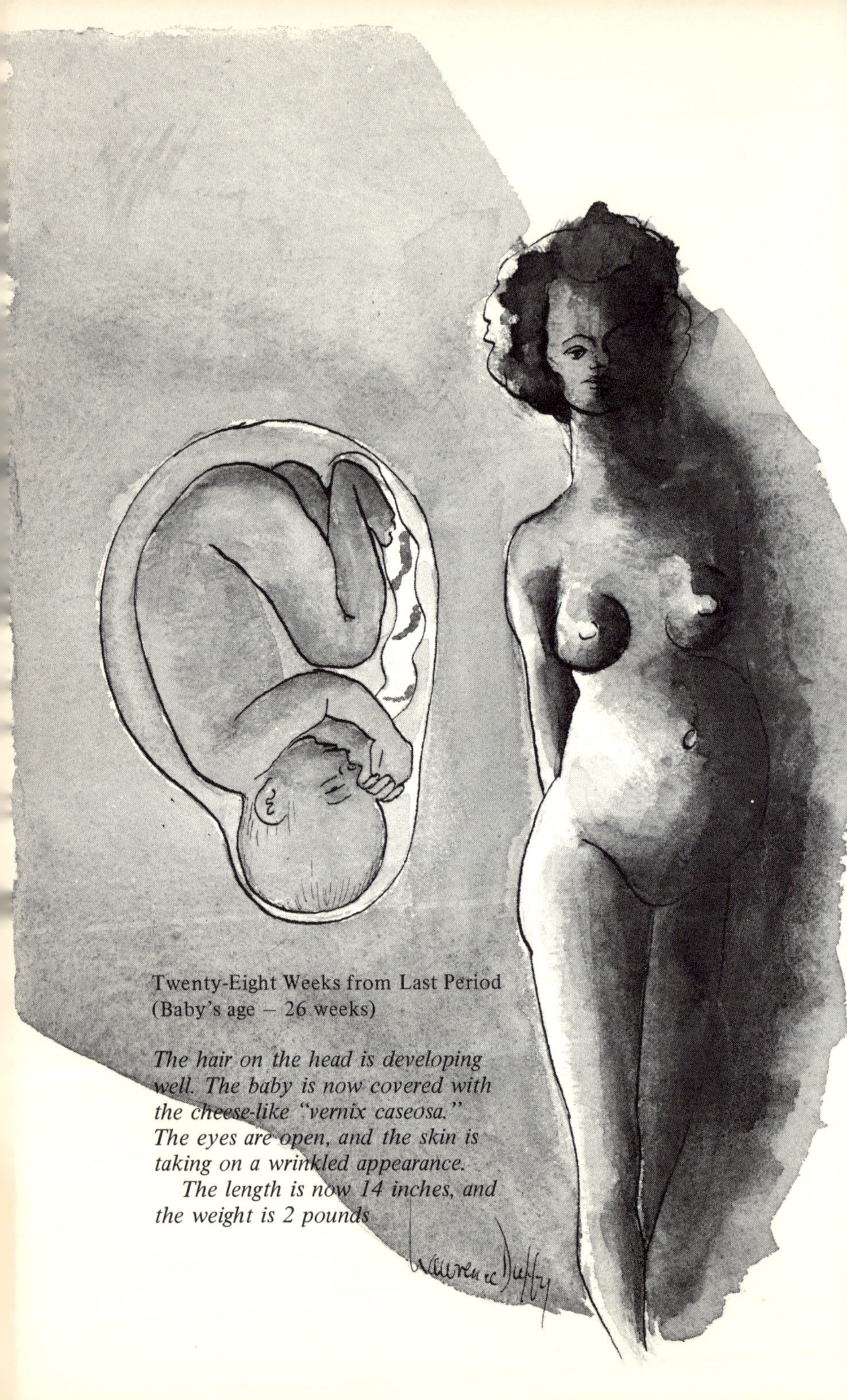

Twenty-Eight Weeks from Last Period
(Baby's age — 26 weeks)

The hair on the head is developing well. The baby is now covered with the cheese-like "vernix caseosa." The eyes are open, and the skin is taking on a wrinkled appearance.

The length is now 14 inches, and the weight is 2 pounds

SIXTH OFFICE VISIT
IN THE SEVENTH MONTH

progress report, in duplicate

By the time of the sixth office visit, a pregnancy is pretty well stabilized. Most of the radical changes have already taken place, the woman has adjusted herself to one surprise after another, and she's usually entitled to face her last two and a half months feeling pretty adept at her management of the reproductive process.

How are you doing?

For many women, the weight budget is pretty bleak at this time. The gain may already have reached the limit, yet there are still two and a half months to go. In such a bind it can be very discouraging to learn that the baby weighs only two and a half pounds at most, and must gain another five pounds or so before birth.

As the uterus rises out of the pelvis a mysterious phenomenon occurs: it rises to the *right* (dextrorotation). Almost invariably this takes place. It is why all pregnant women seem to be a little off center when viewed from the front. No study has revealed the anatomical reason for this piece of trivia. Really!

Earlier, in talking about the importance of weight control, we touched on the condition called toxemia of pregnancy. This is the time it may begin to show itself. At this examination the doctor is especially watchful for any of the three conditions that usually precede the disease: excess weight, swelling, and high blood pressure.

We can't say that these conditions cause the disease; but they are nearly always present in women who develop toxemia. Because weight and fluid control are especially significant now, it is important that any pregnant woman know something about toxemia.

The word "toxemia" indicates that the patient suffers from a toxin, in this case one that is produced by the pregnancy. This is probably true, but any candid medical man must admit that we haven't yet found what that toxin is.

One of the reasons that the search has been fruitless is that there seems to be no way to reproduce the disease in any test animal. The whole range of materials found in toxemia has been introduced into all sorts of animals, but there has never been one that has developed a disease like human toxemia.

This is apparently an affliction that strikes homo sapiens—women only. Since we don't know what causes it, and since we can't duplicate it in any other species, it remains a mystery.

We are fairly certain that whatever causes toxemia of pregnancy is probably produced in the placenta, passing into the mother's circulatory system and raising all kinds of havoc. Placental function is blamed because toxemia almost always clears up shortly after delivery, when the placenta has passed out of the body.

Just before toxemia becomes acute, we may see a sudden increase in the three conditions that pregnant women are told to keep under control. The first increase is in weight. With it comes greater swelling of the ankles and puffiness in the hands, neck and face. This suggests that fluid balance has altered radically. There will probably also be a significant rise in blood pressure.

Doctors are currently somewhat frustrated in their approach to this danger. Traditionally we have tried to hold down weight gain, eliminate excess fluid by various means, and lower blood pressure.

But recently new research suggests that these measures may no longer be regarded as medical gospel. Enforced weight loss may impede the baby's development; diuretic medication to eliminate fluid may have an adverse effect upon the mother; and even the old canon about salt control may fail to eliminate the cause of this mysterious affliction.

I still feel that excess weight is bad; I will continue to tell my patients to cut down on salt intake; and I will use the best methods known to cope with fluid retention. These steps may not overcome the threat of toxemia altogether, as previously thought, but at least I can be confident that they keep the patient far more comfortable. And no one in medicine will deny that toxemia of pregnancy is seldom, if ever, seen where weight, fluids and salt are under good control.

What is especially unfortunate is that most women who approach toxemia are those who are not under regular prenatal care, therefore we don't see them until the disease has become acute.

In a woman who is checked regularly, the presence of the ominous signals means that her doctor can exercise control over her food, fluids and salt. Sometimes, a woman who has practiced excellent self-discipline finds that the metabolism of her pregnancy suddenly goes wild, and before she knows it, she is in trouble. This is extremely rare. In private practice fewer than one out of 100 women develop toxemia.

But what about those women who are not seen by a doctor regularly during their pregnancy? We like to think, in this country, that good care is available to all, and in most places it is. Yet we have not educated women to its importance. Even where such care is free, there are many women who do not take advantage of it because they are not aware of its benefits. The warning signs of impending toxemia are not known to them, so they continue life as usual until the disease becomes severe and dangerous.

For example, a major indicator of toxemia is the presence of albumin in the urine. A woman under regular care has a sample of her urine tested every month; if albumin is found, appropriate action can be taken. The woman without care has no clue that something has gone wrong.

Too late she begins to react to the painful symptoms: wicked headache, abdominal pain and blurred vision. Unfortunately, by the time these symptoms are discovered, gross damage may already have been done. The kidneys are especially vulnerable; a woman who has gone this far into toxemia is not only endangered by the disease itself, but her kidneys may have been permanently damaged.

Prolonged toxemia directly threatens the mother's future health. But what about the child? We know that a baby born too early will face terrible challenges to its survival.

The decision is difficult, and every hour changes the prospects. Ultimately there is no choice, for soon the baby's life will be menaced by the grave illness of its mother. They must be separated. But this is not an insensitive decision, for it throws the odds against the survival of the child.

The situation is not altogether stark. Toxemia can almost always be dealt with. Simple bed rest usually works wonders, so the patient may be brought into the hospital. There are proper medicines available to bring her blood pressure under control.

A woman who has toxemia but no other complicating conditions can usually be managed toward successful delivery. But any pre-existing kidney disease places the toxemic patient's future into jeopardy. If she is to avoid this hazard it may be necessary to deliver her regardless of the immaturity of the child.

Toxemia superimposed on pre-existing kidney disease can cause such damage to the mother as to preclude her bearing any more children and to shorten her own life expectancy. Both participants in the birth are thus victims of the dreadful prospects of this disease.

This scary exposition may be painful but is justified if only it will persuade a pregnant reader who has not put herself in a doctor's care to do so without delay.

Good prenatal care is generally available everywhere, including communities where women cannot afford to pay for it. Unfortunately, a woman may be ignorant or fearful of it, she may have family or transportation problems, or she may simply not understand how important it is for her to be seen regularly. This is why large city hospitals find that despite the availability of free prenatal care, 25 per cent of the women admitted have already developed toxemia and are vulnerable to the sad results. About 1,000 of these women die of the disease each year, which is disheartening enough by itself. But added to that is the loss of 30,000 babies a year due to neglected toxemia in the mothers.

This is the place for me to expound a bit on my feeling that eventually the large problems in medicine will not be solved by the Department of Health, Education, and Welfare, but rather by the Department of Transportation. We must stop duplicating the esoterics of medicine in every village and hamlet just to satisfy the egos of various chiefs of services. This drives the cost of medicine ever upward. Instead there should be a way of quickly moving the seriously ill to a core (even if distant) hospital that can take care of unusual complications that may arise. In other words, bring the outlying patient to the hospital rather than the hospital to the patient.

Now a word here about a new concept in medicine, the physician's assistant, and an old concept in obstetrics, the midwife. In areas where there are no doctors to monitor patients, the physician's assistant can be invaluable in spotting the seriously ill, the complicated case, the case needing the supervision of a trained specialist. This is no more evident than in the field of obstetrics. There are areas in this country without adequate numbers of physicians—these areas are ripe for paramedical personnel, and for midwives who can handle prenatal care and uncomplicated deliveries. The problem is the difficult case—that is where transportation to a center for medical expertise is of the essence.

Midwifery is becoming increasingly popular as more and more women wish to be in the hands of female attendants. A concept which in blighted areas is a necessity is becoming acceptable even in areas where there is an overabundance of obstetricians. This is not a plea for midwives to take over our work, but it is a plea for understanding the wishes and needs of some women to be cared for by other women. Also, in deprived urban areas that are physician-poor, a well-trained midwife may be the saving grace for pregnant clinic patients.

I am not an advocate of delivery at home. I believe too deeply that the advantages of what a hospital has to offer — a blood bank, proper anesthesia, adequate numbers of assisting hands, etc., make delivery much safer for mother and baby. But to satisfy the needs of some women who wish to have their babies within the family milieu, some hospitals are forming "alternative rooms" in which the labor presided over by a midwife may be conducted with the husband and other members of the family present. The important plus for this patient is that even though she may be satisfying some of her psychological needs, she is just down the hall from all that medical science has to offer her and her baby if the need should arise.

Even hospitals that have not as yet instituted the alternative method have greatly relaxed their rules about husbands and children visiting mother before and after delivery. The total family involvement is slowly but surely being brought to fruition. Women's needs in childbirth are changing, and sensitive hospitals are changing too. I want to see it all accomplished, but I want to see it accomplished without sacrificing the monumental advances that have been made toward the safety of the laboring mother-to-be, and her valuable package.

After so dire a consideration as toxemia, other afflictions of late pregnancy may seem trivial. But these bothersome conditions are uncomfortable enough to warrant attention.

Insomnia, for instance. If anyone deserves sleep it is a woman who is toting an increasingly heavy package around with her. Yet it happens that many women find sound sleep ever harder to come by as they advance toward term.

The most common reason is that they just can't get comfortable in bed. You'll hear a lot about the efficiency of the package that contains the baby, but its wrapping makes it no less cumbersome.

Pregnancy exerts stresses and strains everywhere. Muscles and joints may get tired or sore as the day progresses, so that you find yourself to be a system of aches and pains when you get into bed. If you're lucky enough to locate a relaxed position, it seems to last only a few minutes; then a limb will begin to tingle from poor circulation, or an internal part will begin to hurt, and you are forced to thrash around seeking another moderately tolerable sleeping position.

Another common cause of sleeplessness is a baby who seems to belong to the night people. Though most women become accustomed to moderate fetal action at night, some babies are so restless and energetic that they seem to be deliberately keeping Mama awake for company. You'd think at least such babies would have the decency to kick in rhythm, but they don't; every jolt may come as a surprise.

A very effective treatment for persistent sleeplessness in late pregnancy is to end the day with a leisurely soak in a hot bath. This will help to relax the tired muscles, take the strain off sore joints and, who knows, it may also quiet down the internal performer.

Of course, there are sleeping pills, and the idea of taking them is often tempting. But they should be resorted to only with specific permission of the doctor—who will probably be quite reluctant to prescribe them. We have discovered that sleep is a fairly complicated process, consisting of differing levels that must be gone through and returned from systematically. Medication can produce sleep, but it may also upset the sequence of passage through these levels, producing problems that persist beyond the temporary insomnia.

For example, a period of relying upon sleeping pills may result in nightmares after the pills are given up. These dreams can be terrifying by themselves. They'll awaken the former pill-taker and prevent her from getting back to sleep. Her temptation is to return to the pills, but this only ingrains the dependency. The natural process of sleep becomes further disturbed, and shortly the pills fail to do their job unless the dosage is increased. Recovery from a pill-induced sleep imbalance is far more difficult than trying to exercise some degree of control over the temporary sleeplessness that sometimes occurs.

Another inconvenience of pregnancy, particularly in the last half, is nasal congestion and nosebleed. The congestion results from the increased sensitivity of mucous membrane. Since there is greatly increased blood supply to this tissue, the ordinary irritations of the nasal lining are more likely to break small blood vessels. The bleeding doesn't usually last long, but it's a nuisance.

Women who have persistent nosebleeds while pregnant are often given a mixture of menthol in oil with which to lubricate the nasal lining once or twice a day.

Nosebleeds or not, many women react to the increased activity in the mucosa by feeling as though they are going through the entire period with a head cold. Their noses are stuffy, sinuses are blocked, and their ears seem to pop all day long. This is called "allergic rhinitis of pregnancy." There are nose drops to relieve it, but there is also a hitch: the condition can easily be overtreated, so the patient never really knows if she's troubled more by the treatment than by the condition itself.

If all of the gloom contained in this chapter suggests that pregnancy is a pretty deplorable method of producing children, consider something that might be worse: to undergo the symptoms of pregnancy without being pregnant at all.

This condition is called pseudocyesis, which means false pregnancy. One of the amazing experiences of obstetrics is to treat a woman whose mind and body have tricked her into believing that she has conceived a child, and to find that there's nothing there.

It's not necessarily a human fluke, either. Pseudocyesis is sometimes found among animals; cats, dogs, cows and horses have been known to go through the same sort of sham maternity.

The main reason that cases of human false pregnancy can become so convincing is that the victims usually stay away from doctors during the early months. Thus a woman may miss several menstrual periods, and finally arrive in a doctor's office wearing maternity clothes and with her abdomen impressively inflated. She will also describe a whole sequence of symptoms related to pregnancy.

Invariably, such a woman will emphasize her "morning sickness."

Consciously or otherwise, she makes her body resort to this most impressive "proof" that she has conceived. In complete irrationality, however, she may insist that she couldn't possibly be pregnant, or refuse to discuss it, yet continue with her charade of symptoms.

But cursory physical examination very quickly reveals the delusion. For there is no enlargement of the uterus, a pregnancy urine test is negative, and the abdominal protrusion is ultimately identified for what it actually is—nothing but gas!

Psychiatrists have found all sorts of causes behind this strange defiance of Nature. A girl may be trying to spite a domineering father. Or she may feel so guilty about having had intercourse that she unconsciously makes her body punish itself. Or she may wish so fervently for a love fulfillment that she'll attempt to produce its physical results. Once in a while a woman can do this despite the fact that she has had no intimacy with a man!

There are undoubtedly many early false pregnancies that are "deflated" by the simple announcement that a laboratory test shows the woman is not pregnant. When a woman misses periods and doesn't know that she's trying to fool herself—and most often she doesn't—she might decide to check the possibility of pregnancy by visiting a doctor. Since thousands of women miss periods, suspect conception, and check it out this way, we have no idea how many might have started fantasy pregnancies and then abandoned them on facing the unalterable evidence that there is no embryo within them.

But among those who do not seek medical confirmation, the self-delusion can become spectacular. The patient's breasts may enlarge and harden. Her intestines will not only become distended, but the bulge can be confined to the region where it is most impressive.

For the obstetrician, such cases can be difficult to handle. He can simply tell the woman bluntly, "You are not pregnant." But this takes no account of her sensibilities. He can pretend to be unaware that anything such as fantasy pregnancy exists and give her several plausible reasons why she mistakenly thought she had conceived. If she is a patient of long acquaintance, he may choose to deliver the entire truth—that some unconscious drive within her has become so powerful that it has interrupted the normal functions of her body, and that she therefore may need psychiatric help. Whichever approach is used, the effect usually solves the physical problem. The shock may linger on, but the symptoms of pregnancy disappear.

Then there are the cases of people who so fervently wish to participate in the pregnancy of a loved one that they duplicate its symptoms in themselves.

It is not at all uncommon for an overprotective mother to become empathetically and even hysterically involved in her daughter's pregnancy. Perhaps due to her own experience, such a mother is able to put her own body through the paces of pregnancy again. It's amazing to learn of or actually see the amount of suffering such women can bring upon themselves. It's as though such a mother is saying, "This poor little girl can't possibly carry that baby all by herself, therefore I must carry it for her."

Don't laugh, for very shortly you are about to have such an experience of helpless empathy with your own baby. At the time your offspring begins to take solid foods, see if you don't catch yourself opening and closing your *own* mouth, as if to help your inexperienced eater to get the food off the spoon. This is exactly what the falsely pregnant grandma-to-be is doing, only on a fantastically more elaborate scale.

The press recently carried a story of identical twin girls in England, one of whom was pregnant. Her nonpregnant sister experienced the full spectrum of pregnancy symptoms, including severe and painful uterine contractions at the time of her twin's labor.

The false labor continued and intensified at home while the truly pregnant twin was engaged in delivery at the hospital. After the baby was born, the new mother got word to her sister that the worst was over. Only then did the nonpregnant twin's contractions cease.

And if you think *that* is weird, what about sympathetic pregnancy in a person who couldn't possibly become pregnant anyway?

Yes, my dear—husbands! Every now and then we hear of men who go through all kinds of discomfort as they empathize madly in behalf of their wives. They'll be nauseous when the wife is nauseous, dizzy when she is dizzy, and may match her, ache for ache. Those of us who see such cases fervently hope that the husband won't be around in the event that his wife's bag of waters breaks at home, for his obvious response might be an embarrassing one!

A strange and wondrous process, this system of producing babies, sometimes even affecting those who can't do it.

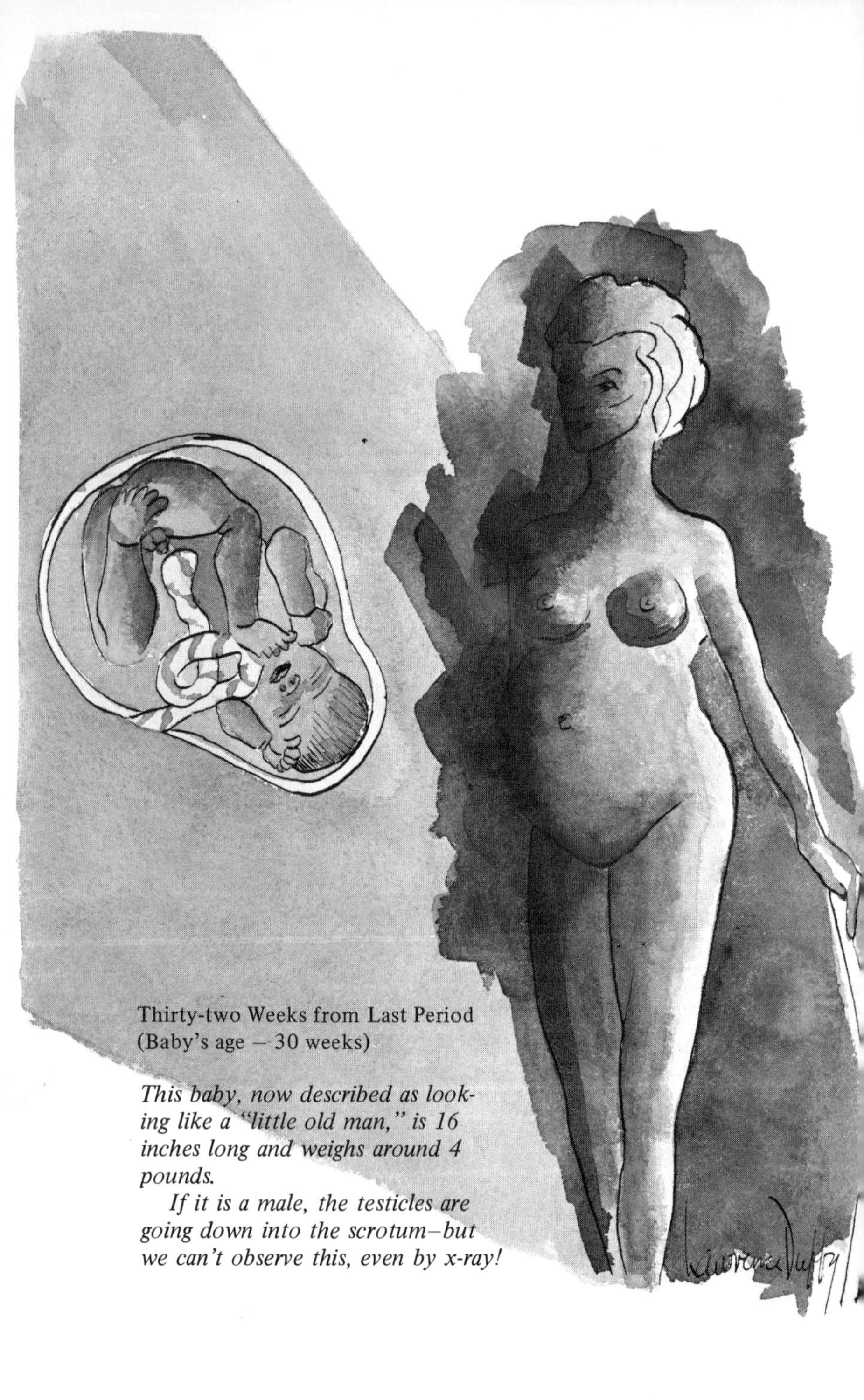

Thirty-two Weeks from Last Period
(Baby's age — 30 weeks)

This baby, now described as looking like a "little old man," is 16 inches long and weighs around 4 pounds.

If it is a male, the testicles are going down into the scrotum—but we can't observe this, even by x-ray!

SEVENTH OFFICE VISIT
IN THE EIGHTH MONTH
"ridin' high"

By the time of the seventh office visit, your uterus extends about four finger breadths above your navel. It will go a bit higher, and further enlargement laterally will make the burden more cumbersome.

The added weight has undoubtedly already produced its problems: shortness of breath, displaced balance, sore joints and fatigue.

Your body seems like an occupied village; the enemy may be friendly, but his presence produces a grossly overcrowded situation.

Nevertheless, if a woman has kept to her diet and is walking properly she may appear quite attractive at this stage. Few women believe it, but there is a whole corps of males who find pregnant women to have a special sort of feminine allure. They are the ones you're likely to see dancing with pregnant women at parties where other men regard an expectant mother as though her abdomen contained not a baby but an imminent catastrophe.

A pregnant woman's tendency is usually to brand such gestures as gallant or merciful. This is unnecessarily modest at a time when a little vanity can be helpful. Why not flatly acknowledge that your pregnancy might just make you so radiant and alluring that you have turned these gentlemen on?

For we have it on the best of authority—from men—that it is perfectly possible that a woman can be pregnant and sexy at the same time.

Some women report that their husband's ardor seems to increase proportionately to the size of their abdominal bulge. Such men are forever grabbing a quick kiss, or patting the protuberance, or hugging in spite of the barrier. If the woman happens to be one who believes that she has never looked worse in her life, perhaps her best philosophy comes from the credo of the hippies:

"Whatever turns you on, Baby!"

In a world as obviously well planned as ours it would be outrageous if the female of the species, so assiduously sought after by the male for purposes of mating and reproduction, should so lose her glamour in the process that she becomes no more alluring than a pail full of chicken feet. In the animal kingdom, males are increasingly protective and thoughtful of their mates toward the time when their young will be born. Humans are not much different, despite the fact that their females feel that nothing about them is visible except the portable mountain.

There's no denying, however, that the baby by now has become an impressive package. It is now large enough to be pretty much committed to its most favorable position for delivery—head down and rump forward, pitched a little to one side or the other. You can probably tell if this is the case by feeling various parts of your abdomen.

When a baby is properly positioned at this stage it is not likely to shift around. Only a small percentage of babies remain feet first in the eighth month, and most of these finally right themselves before term. The statistics run that about 97 per cent of all births are head-first presentations. Many of the three per cent in breech respond to manipulation at delivery, and obstetricians are specially trained to manage delivery of those babies who insist on doing it the hard way.

The doctor determines the position of the baby by palpating the woman's abdomen, and confirms it by the location of the fetal heartbeat. If the baby's back is up against the front wall of the uterus, that's where the strongest heartbeat will be heard, because the sound is conducted through the bones of the baby's shoulders and back.

The best sound may be heard to the left or right of the midline, indicating that the baby faces one side or the other. Later, the descent of the baby deeper into the pelvis can be determined by the change in the location of the site where the heartbeat is best heard. It's much like finding the best place in a room for listening to music in stereo.

If the baby is in breech position, the heartbeat will be heard much higher up, usually above the navel, because that's where the bones of the shoulders and back will be pressing.

However, in the eighth month the baby is still small enough to be mobile inside the uterus, and nearly all the natural pressures and movements tend to direct the head downward. The shape of the uterus itself helps to nudge the head downward. Nature has her way most often. When she doesn't, your obstetrician is there to save her reputation.

The baby at this time is about 16 inches long and is usually described as looking "like a little old man." No instructor in obstetrics whom I have ever encountered describes it as looking like a little old woman, which may be another of life's injustices. The skin is red and wrinkled, and its weight is a few ounces under four pounds.

It is interesting to note that racial characteristics are fairly indistinguishable all the way along through pregnancy. This is especially true of color, for all babies are "baby color" rather than the color of their parents. Pigmentation comes along after birth.

If the baby is male, the testicles may have just recently descended into the scrotum.

A child born at 30 weeks has a slightly better than even chance to survive, but expert and intensive care is required.

There's a superstition that a child born before term will be healthier and more beautiful than one born on schedule, but there is no scientific basis for such a belief. The story probably derived from the fact that odds for survival of such an early birth were formerly so unfavorable that children who made it were looked upon in wonder.

But the legend persists stubbornly that early babies are superior, and denying it again here isn't likely to change things. In any healthy pregnancy, the nearer a child is to term, the greater are its chances of being normal and strong. Dramatic births, in which the child overcomes terrifying threats, tend to be remembered and recounted by parents, who invariably begin, "You'd never guess it to look at him now, but. . . . ." It makes for a gripping story, but there is quiet satisfaction in an incident-free birth, despite the fact that it may not give you as much to talk about. And your child will greatly appreciate it later.

All through this book the tacit assumption has been that the woman who is seeking information about her pregnancy is married and is carrying a baby she wants that has been fathered by her husband. This is a most convenient situation, much to be desired, but of course, it doesn't always apply.

*Un*married women get pregnant too.

Married women sometimes conceive with men who are not their husbands.

And wives are not universally delighted by the news that they have a developing child within them.

These are complications which in no way disqualify such women from handling pregnancy as intelligently as those who are sailing along happily.

They deserve special consideration, which is given here for the fairly arbitrary reason that, at 30 weeks, pregnancy is just about impossible to conceal.

During the time that socially complicated pregnancies are not visible, many of these women go along without any medical guidance at all. Some may have taken a test to verify pregnancy, but after that they are inclined to keep the fact to themselves as they try to reach a decision on the best course of action to take.

It is an unhappy fact of our society that we have established moral rules that make the medical problem secondary to the problem of "What will people think?" This is a source of constant frustration to physicians; for regardless of their field of specialization, they keep running across cases of women whose lives have been made miserable because they are pregnant when society dictates that they are not supposed to be, or when they themselves don't want to be. To make it worse, we don't hear about them until some dreadful complication, social or medical, has flared up.

Obstetricians expect to be consulted in confidence about such sexual accidents because they relate directly to their field. But appeals for help and advice are also made to pathologists, internists, surgeons, allergists, psychiatrists—in fact, anybody associated with medicine.

But hardly ever do the calls come soon enough.

A doctor is not entitled to make any moral judgments whatever about someone who comes to him with a problem of inconvenient pregnancy. His function is to offer medical service, regardless of circumstance.

If a man mangles a hand while trying to blow a safe open, it is our job to repair it, not to tell him he got what he deserved for being a thief. By the same ethics, we are not allowed to cluck disapproval over any woman's sexual caprices.

Nevertheless, there it is; society professes to deplore pregnancy outside of marriage or pregnancy by the wrong partner within marriage. We make pregnancy evidence per se of wrongdoing, and punish the carrier accordingly.

This book makes no such judgment. The fact of the pregnancy entitles a woman to medical advice and help. But the habit of society to brand certain pregnancies as illicit leads the victims to concealment, and this often results in serious medical problems.

Therefore let's consider the unlucky woman who is more occupied with her problem of being pregnant in a society that disapproves than she is as a woman who needs medical guidance: It is quite late for her, at 30 weeks, but she still has several choices of action.

One avenue that by now is definitely closed, however, is abortion, because it must be done long before this time. In advanced pregnancy there are complications which make abortion dangerous under the best of conditions. No responsible physician would consider an abortion at six months into the pregnancy.

Let's consider the plight of a woman who cannot take advantage of legal abortion. Remember, lack of money and distance from the facilities are not the only considerations. She may be pregnant by a partner other than her husband; or she may be a girl still under the roof and authority of her parents. If she is to be aborted, it must be done during the short period of time that will arouse no one's suspicions. This is why a woman's first option—to end the pregnancy—deteriorates so rapidly. Most often she doesn't suspect that she has conceived until she misses her first period, which is at least fourteen days after the intercourse that scored. She will then probably allow herself a week or ten days in the hope that "her friend" will arrive. When menstruation does not occur, she may lose a few more days in deciding on a pregnancy test and waiting for its result. After that, because the idea of abortion is not an easy one for most women to accept, several more days may pass before she determines to take action.

The major attraction of abortion is obvious: the problem of the baby is instantly eliminated. For many women, the incident ends right there. This is especially true if the woman can obtain her abortion before anyone but herself and confidantes become aware that she was pregnant.

But in the panicky contemplation of abortion hardly anybody considers the long-term effects, such as guilt, shame, revulsion and regret. I am not moralizing; there are deep-seated emotional forces which can cause some women far more grief than would delivering an illegitimate child.

The last few years have produced revolutionary social and legal changes that have made early abortion acceptable. In January 1973, the United States Supreme Court wiped out all state laws restricting abortions.

In so doing, the Court was not saying that abortions could now be *done*—they had always been *done*. But most of them had been done badly, and at great cost to the patient. What the Court said was that abortions were now *legal*, which meant that they could now be done *properly*.

Until that decision, even the hardiest of women found the abortion experience to be one of shock, expense, and danger. Most patients had no idea of the conditions they would encounter in the process, or the methods used. Some techniques were crude and brutal. The operator might try to irrigate the uterus with an astringent solution, which could be terribly dangerous. Such a solution may permanently damage tissue; the pressure of its flow may cause emboli; bacteria can be introduced to start infection.

Another method was to pack the uterus with gauze, with the intent of causing contractions to expel the foreign object, and the embryo along with it. Here the dangers were damage to the cervix in the packing process and infection from non-sterile materials and instruments.

The quack abortionist might simply introduce a rubber catheter into the cervix and leave it there, waiting for abortion to occur as the body attempted to eject it. This was quite painful and included a high hazard of infection, since the catheter might have to be in place for several days.

Only because abortion was taken out of the hands of physicians and prevented as a matter of law were these methods able to wreak such a heavy toll on women. Even if the abortionist happened to possess medical skills, the fact that he or she worked outside the law precluded proper medical care.

Any woman ought to have a clear idea of what must be done to her body in order to rid it of an established pregnancy.

The safest method commonly used is dilating the cervix until its opening is large enough for a curette or a suction tip to pass through. This requires a good deal of medical training and a rather high level of professional skill. The later in the pregnancy that abortion is done, the greater is the risk of damage to the uterus. Such injury can seldom be assessed immediately, which is why the patient should be kept under observational care.

Few illegal abortionists could accommodate their clients for any longer time than it takes to do the surgery, so they simply told them to go home and get into bed.

Now that physicians, hospitals, and clinics may perform abortions openly, most of the incompetent and unqualified practitioners have been forced out of their bloody business.

Before the Court's decision, the figures from any municipal hospital offering emergency treatment showed a dreadful number of abortion cases that went wrong: infections, hemorrhages, permanent loss of childbearing capability, and death.

Within existing law: In the first trimester *no one* can interfere in a woman's decision for abortion. Neither the state or the government can tell her she can't have an abortion, only that it must be done by an M.D.

In the 3rd trimester the state can insist that the abortion be done only to protect the life (read "health, either physical or mental") of the mother. But for all practical purposes abortions are not done if the fetus to be aborted is capable of living outside the protective atmosphere of the womb.

Where properly performed abortion is most needed, and where

it would spare the most grief, is among people who are so poor that they not only can't afford it, they don't even know it is available.

Abortion is still very much in the news. It is a hotly controversial subject in which the right of the bearer is pitted against the right of the borne. Many insist upon the principle that a woman be allowed to control her own body; others demand that the status of human-ness be granted at the moment of conception.

There is an abundance of evidential support for both sides of the argument. But the principal result of the discussion has been to make the decision on abortion largely one that the woman considering it must make alone. She may receive advice and persuasion from her lover, her family, her clergyman, and her physician. But ultimately, the choice falls solely upon herself.

Anything further that I might say on the abortion decision would necessarily fall into the category of persuasive advice, and mine would not be any more helpful than anyone else's. But I will freely advise on advice: I would urge any woman facing the choice to inform herself as fully as possible on all phases of her decision: ethics, ecology, health, psychology, and the personal desires of everyone involved. Only then will the decision be intelligent. But even then, it will not be easy.

As humans we have the ability and the need to reproduce, but unfortunately we don't have the sense of responsibility to reproduce only out of love. Therefore unwanted pregnancies occur. Even though birth control may be assiduously used, we know it to be imperfect. Laws may be passed that would forbid abortions, but no law has ever been devised that can prevent abortions from being done. Pregnant women, aided and abetted by their inseminators, will be forced back into the shady world of the illegal, the unclean, the costly and the degrading. No one who supports abortion as part of the freedom of choice for women in any way supports forced termination of pregnancy--but for those women who feel the need, that choice must be available under the best medical circumstances and at a price that does not make second-class citizens out of the economically disadvantaged.

After the opportunity of choosing abortion has passed, a woman must deal with herself as one who will go on to deliver her baby, adjusting herself to the judgments of society as best she can.

Here she has several options: She can marry the man who made her pregnant. She can marry a man whom she has made *think* he made her pregnant. Or she can marry a man who is willing to bail her out even though he has never touched her—and you'd be amazed at the number of such gallant souls there are.

In each of these possibilities she is more likely to be bending under the dictates of society than doing what she really wants to do. For the sad fact is that though good marriages produce babies, babies do not necessarily produce good marriages.

Such unions, as in the case of abortion, often turn out to be an immediate answer, but not a permanent solution.

This is why many women rule out both abortion and marriage to deal with the baby on other terms. For there are still several choices:

A pregnant girl can decide to deliver the baby and give it up for adoption. She can keep the baby and tell society to be damned. Or she can find a secret haven for her child until such time as her life can be adjusted to accommodate its presence without stigma.

In most of the charitable homes that offer care for unmarried pregnant girls, a strong persuasive effort is made to have the girl give the child up for adoption. There are still enough childless couples who want children for most white babies to be spoken for before they are born.

For black and mixed-race children, the prospects are not so rosy. Racial discrimination is still so strong that it has prevented such childless couples from reaching the level of economic independence needed to make adoption possible.

According to the arguments of racists, black women are charged not only with being promiscuous, but with having an indifferent regard for the children they may bear outside of marriage. But the fact is that ghetto women have limited access to birth control methods, and so are more vulnerable to pregnancy. And furthermore, it is among unmarried black women that the choice is most often made to keep the baby and give it a home. The decision is usually accepted as readily by the woman's family as by herself. The black community embraces such arrangements as a joint responsibility, placing no moral judgment upon mother or child.

This practice has been widely and heartlessly misinterpreted by much of the white community. They say that women in the ghettos keep having these babies because each one produces another welfare allotment. But the stipend received is never generous enough to cover the costs of raising the child. And the accusation fails to take any account whatever of the fact that unmarried black girls who are *not* on welfare also have babies and keep them.

Of all the choices available, this one may have the greatest merit. It recognizes the innocence of the child and attributes maximum importance to the role of the natural mother.

And for those who would pass judgment on what they regard as the immorality of the poor having babies out of wedlock, I would cite the reasonable explanation once offered by the late Richard Cardinal Cushing of Boston: When a lady asked him why it is that in places such as Bolivia (where he maintained extensive missions) where people are poor and downtrodden, "that's where we find the highest birth rate?" he answered, "My dear, there's nothing else for them to do down there!"

Married or unmarried, a woman 30 weeks pregnant has the right to assess herself occasionally, and wonder what ravages the bearing of a child will wreak on her figure.

In our society we happen to place fairly high value on good-looking legs. It is unfortunate that a toll of pregnancy can be the development of varicose veins. Whether or not the veins of her legs are going to stand up under the strain of pregnancy depends pretty much on the patient's heredity. Either she got good valves in her leg veins, or she didn't.

A little basic anatomy is required here: as oxygenated blood leaves the heart, it follows a route of arteries, which are blood vessels that are wide open for unimpeded flow. These arteries keep branching off into smaller and smaller vessels until they finally reach a hair-thin curve known as a capillary loop. From that point on, the blood is on its way back to the heart and lungs through return vessels that are called veins.

Because the thrust of the heartbeat is less strongly exerted, due to the distance from the heart, the blood needs extra help in making its return. For this reason, the veins are equipped with one-way valves. The valves open as the heartbeat pushes the blood through, then close to prevent it from falling back.

In the legs, where the distance from the heart is greatest, these valves are subjected to maximum load. If they happen to be strong and flexible, as is usually the case, they can handle the extra volume and heavier load that is caused by pregnancy.

But if the valves are weak, or sparsely located, the sheer weight of the returning blood can cause the veins to swell. Circulation is sluggish, so the veins become distended and sore.

Varicose veins are usually visible first along the inner sides of the legs and at the back of the knees. They may be felt as a sensation of fatigue, or slight ache. Not much can be done to prevent this varicosity, but the patient can take steps to minimize the enlargement and ease the discomfort.

Once the tendency toward varicosity is discovered, the woman ought to allow herself several arbitrary rest periods during the day. She should lie down with her feet elevated so that her heels are higher than her hips. This makes gravity her ally, because the blood can flow out of the leg veins back toward the heart more easily.

For the times when she must be on her feet, she can help herself by wearing support stockings, or the more rugged elastic stockings, or even by wrapping her legs in Ace bandages.

Any garment worn to prevent varicosity ought to be put on before the leg veins have a chance to become engorged. On awakening, the woman can lie in bed and pull the stockings on with her legs elevated, or wrap the bandages before she stands up.

An exercise that will help stimulate return flow from the legs is the upside down bicycle routine. Lie on the floor, prop your hips up with your hands and rotate the legs vigorously. At 30 weeks, the baby may get in your way, but it won't get seasick.

Varicosities will generally clear up between pregnancies, but they tend to return a little more severely each time a woman carries. Surgical correction is hardly ever advisable during the pregnancy, and it will not prevent other veins from enlarging in the next one. When a woman's childbearing days are over, the enlarged veins can be tied off or injected so that they are no longer bothersome or conspicuous.

It would not be honest to say that exercise, garment support and frequent daily rest will prevent the formation of varicose veins. But these precautions will help significantly and are well worth the time they require.

In the same category as troublesome veins of the legs are those of the rectum which are called hemorrhoids when they enlarge. With the increased pressure of pregnancy in the late months, these veins can swell and become tender. Hard bowel movements cause them to protrude. Because they are exposed and vulnerable, they may bleed and become painful.

Itching and minor pain are indicators that hemorrhoids—or piles—are a possibility, and the best approach is preventive. Supplement the diet with leafy vegetables, salads and coarse cereals. Take a little fruit on going to bed, such as prunes, dates, figs or apples.

Licorice candy will also help, if you can work it into your calorie allowance.

If there is slight bleeding or a bulging anal lump, lubricate the area with a touch of salve containing a local anesthetic. There are several such products available for treatment of hemorrhoids. The swelling and discomfort can also be eased by sitting in a hot tub. But as important as any other treatment is use of the clock; try to put your bowel movements on schedule. If your major evacuation can be had at about the same time each day, unhurried and without straining, you won't be compounding a sensitive condition. Remember that because of the pressure of the birth package, the bowel passage is narrowed, and deserves special consideration to assist its function.

It is interesting to note that neither hemorrhoids nor varicose veins occur in lower animals—this is the price that humans have paid for walking upright rather than on all fours. Women's Lib members may make the most of the fact that females pay the penalty far more frequently than men.

One final note on your condition at 30 weeks: look at your navel. Note that it is now everted, so you can't wear a rhinestone.

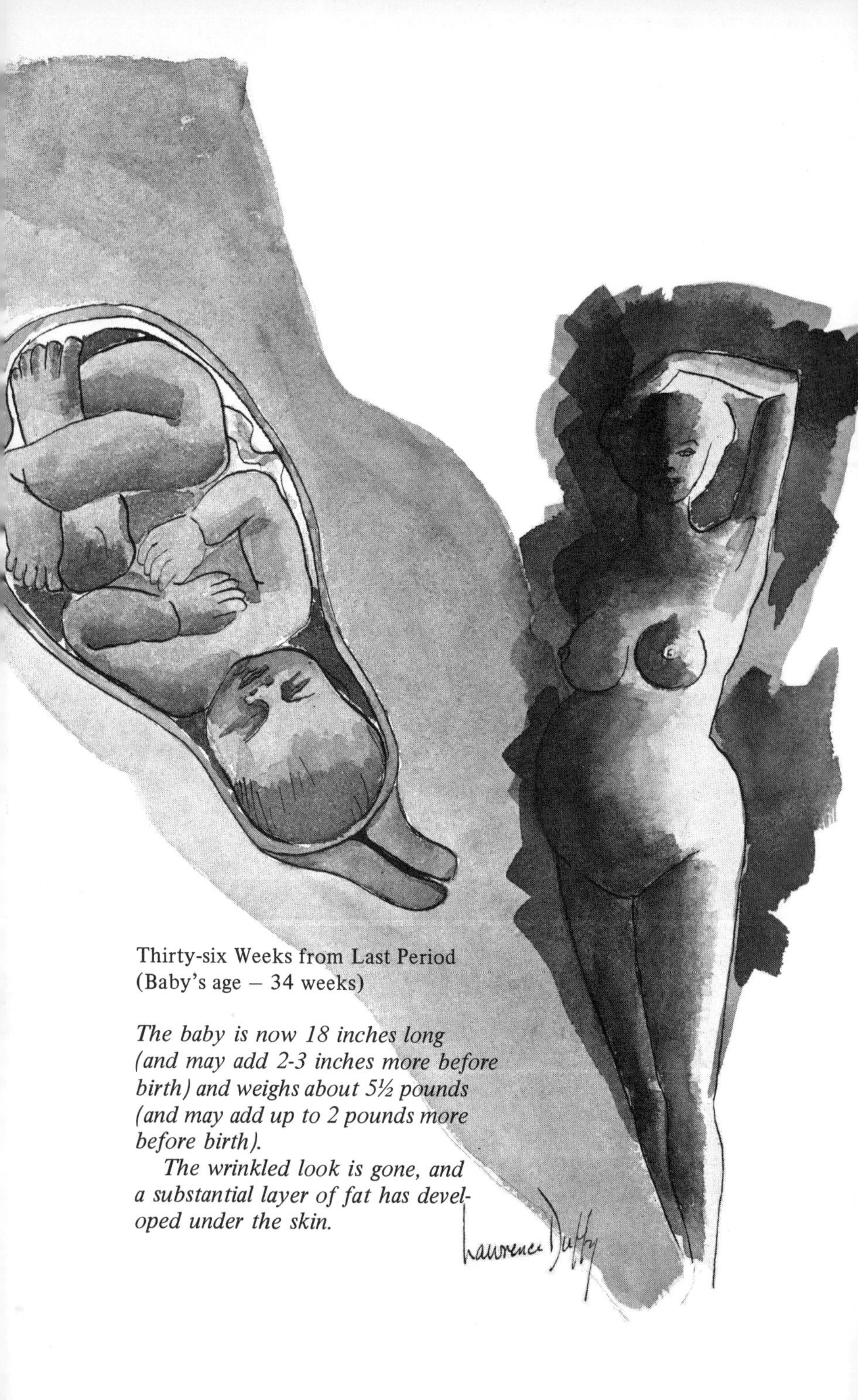

Thirty-six Weeks from Last Period
(Baby's age — 34 weeks)

*The baby is now 18 inches long
(and may add 2-3 inches more before
birth) and weighs about 5½ pounds
(and may add up to 2 pounds more
before birth).*
*The wrinkled look is gone, and
a substantial layer of fat has developed under the skin.*

EIGHTH OFFICE VISIT
IN THE NINTH MONTH
comin' round the mountain

For 34 weeks or so, your baby has been steadily developing toward a degree of maturity and strength that will make possible independent life outside of you. Nine menstrual periods have passed. So why isn't labor just around the corner?

The reason is that you were not pregnant at the time of your last menstrual period. You didn't conceive until two weeks or so later. Now you must wait for the completion of the 267 days that pregnancy generally requires, and that time is still about four weeks away.

Nevertheless, a baby at this stage is in very good shape, and could sustain life without much danger with proper hospital care.

There is still time for significant growth, however. The baby is now about 18 inches long, and may add two or three inches more in length. Its weight is about 5½ pounds, so there is time to accumulate two additional pounds. Since last month the infant has lost the wrinkled look and has probably developed a substantial layer of fat under the skin. This incredible growth machine can be expected to add more weight to its body in the next four weeks than it did during its first six months.

If the mother is Rh-negative, this is the time when the doctor will have another blood sample tested to assure that she has not become sensitized by the blood of an Rh-positive baby. In a first child the probability is that she has not. But if she has had several babies before, and has not received a Rhogam injection after each delivery in which she was found to be free of Rh response, her degree of immunity must be measured to determine how great a threat it poses for the baby.

Where a woman's Rh immunity is high, a method by which the doctor can determine the baby's safety is by taking a sample of the amniotic fluid. Precise measurement of any coloration in the fluid helps the doctor to determine his course of action. He may continue these tests from week to week. If he decides that it will be best to take the baby out of its threatening environment, he may try to induce labor early, or decide to deliver the baby by caesarian section.

But the necessity of such steps can be expected to decrease rapidly as the Rhogam treatment for nonsensitized mothers after each delivery becomes more widely available. A problem that remains is developing a larger source of the Rhogam needed: Rh-negative types who have developed a high level of antibodies against the Rh factor.

There are other situations which might lead a doctor to consider the possibility of early inducement or caesarian section at around the eighth month: toxemia of pregnancy and diabetes. A woman with cardiovascular problems, if she has been brought this far, can probably go on to term.

For most other women, there is little else to do about the tag end of pregnancy except to wait and plan.

Please don't wait and worry. It's just as easy to adopt the attitude that you are now carrying a future President of the United States, possibly the first of her sex to hold the office. Don't bother to memorize the U. S. Constitution, or the speeches of Lincoln, because it will not help to adapt your passenger to the duties of the office. For there is no such thing as prenatal influence.

Once upon a time there was a pregnant woman who was thinking about something else while backing her car out of her driveway, and she slammed into a bakery truck. Three months later her baby was born; on its forehead there was the distinct outline of a Parker House roll!

Baloney!

In the lore of womanhood (new wives as well as old), there are wild and weird tales about the marks placed upon children by prenatal events. "I never ate strawberries in my life, but in my third month, I had a terrible craving for them, so I ate a whole bowl, and broke out in a rash. My baby was born with a strawberry mark on his neck." Or, "Muriel was frightened by a snake at a picnic, and when her baby was born, it had a dark, wiggly line down its stomach."

Knockwurst!

On a slightly artier level, some women sincerely believe that they ought to hear classical music while pregnant, visit art galleries, and read good poetry, thus rendering their unborn children more sensitive to life's finer treasures. The truth is that no child becomes a genius because his mother walked under the Harvard arch that says "Veritas," and no child becomes a painter because his mother took him, in utero, through the Louvre.

The myth of prenatal influence can be traced to a rare medical phenomenon: once in a while a woman will suffer a severe emotional or physical shock during her first three months of pregnancy. If such shock produces a sudden lowering of blood pressure, the supply of oxygenated blood to her child may be suddenly reduced. If the drop in blood pressure is drastic, and if, at that precise moment, a formative cell division happens to be taking place in the embryo, the cell division may be damaged and the child can be defective. But this is not only an exceedingly rare event, it is one that never can be proved to have occurred anyway.

Neither can a child's emotional make-up be influenced by events that take place while it is in the womb. In clinging to the belief that such prenatal effect is real, women misinterpret the evidence. Women speak of children who become nervous because their mothers were jittery all through the pregnancy. What they overlook is the fact that the mother probably didn't stop being jittery after the child was born, and that she communicated the trait to her offspring by example. Similarly, it is less reasonable to believe that the characteristic of aggressiveness could have been contained in a gene from the father than that the child learned belligerence from living with an aggressive man.

The transmittable traits that are sent along in the brief moment of conception are altogether physical. The genes carry the keys for the color of eyes and hair, shape of the mouth, relative size of the ears, and tendency toward freckling or darkening in the sun. Some genes tend to dominate, as we see in the preponderance of Rh-positive babies over Rh-negative. A marked facial resemblance between father and son may result from such a dominance.

I know a lawyer who has an unmistakably distinctive speaking voice. When I telephoned his office recently, I heard the same, unusual voice on the line. But it turned out I was hearing the man's oldest son who had just passed the bar and entered practice with his father. Heredity? Or influence? I don't know.

Some very interesting work is being done which suggests that unexpected talents and inclinations may be passed along in the genes. For example, it has been shown that many birds are born already knowing how to sing the song of their species. So perhaps some human babies arrive well prepared to be as stubborn about food as their fathers are. Certainly most parents are prepared to believe that each of their children was born with his own peculiar behavior pattern, pre-programmed and unchangeable by influence.

But remember the other birds—those who can't sing a single note correctly until they hear it from Momma and Poppa.

You can take your choice between inherited and acquired characteristics. But don't try to manipulate them during pregnancy. A genetic declaration was made at the time of conception. It's a little late to try to tinker with it now.

So far as the unborn child's mind is concerned, I believe it comes to consciousness entirely blank. Whatever goes into it and however it ultimately performs are determined by the events to which it is witness. The argument as to whether talent is inherited or developed is a classical one. Fortunately, that debate does not involve obstetricians.

Something else that ought to be dispelled is the concept of "the fragile pregnancy," especially one that has entered its final months. You are not a wounded butterfly, and there is no reason to behave like one or to be treated like one.

Pregnant women are usually young women; in our modern society young women are required to move around. The very fact of expecting a baby often makes it necessary for the family to find bigger quarters. Shifting a household from one place to another involves plenty of physical work, but there is no medical reason why a woman should be timid about doing it.

If move you must, when is the best time? My dear, you may go when it is convenient for you to go. If the move is to be local, just pack up your goods and move. It might be wise to take into account that pregnant women often have bursts of unbelievable energy, and that you might therefore be tempted to do everything yourself. Women have a very powerful nesting instinct which sometimes drives them to overwork in preparation for a new baby. But about the only result is fatigue, especially if the work is done with a baby as big as yours at 34 weeks or so.

Moving a great distance poses other problems; you may have to arrange for a new doctor and a different hospital in which to deliver. Obviously it will be best if all this can be taken care of early, so that you'll be settled down and somewhat at home before reaching the stage in which labor might commence.

But the trip itself is no danger.

The place for a pregnant woman is at home. She shouldn't be gallivanting all over the place. And she certainly shouldn't take long trips.

Rubbish!

How could we possibly have pioneered this country, if pregnant women also had not withstood the bumps and bangs of a prairie schooner? There was a baby born on the *Mayflower,* and thousands of others were carried, steerage class, by pregnant women en route here from the Old World.

In World War II, Korea and Vietnam, brides have traveled all over the world in all kinds of conveyances. They have shown that movement from place to place puts no special strain on pregnancy. Inevitably, we can look forward to the first child to be born weightless in outer space, and I have complete confidence that its mother will withstand the force of lift-off.

Expectant women, the *New England Journal of Medicine* has reported, are remarkably portable.

All that travel requires is common sense, which is somehow abundantly found among pregnant women. Avoid long hauls with too many miles between rest stops. (Your now limited bladder capacity will determine the stops, anyway.) Allow time for nourishing meals, leisurely eaten, and make it a point to get some moderate exercise before piling yourself back into the car.

Should a pregnant woman drive? Why not, if there's space enough for her to get behind the wheel. The more or less fixed posture required of a driver, however, is likely to tire her.

A woman prone to motion sickness can fend it off with the modern medications for that purpose. These have no adverse effect upon the baby. Neither does the motion, for the baby is bobbing around contentedly in its sea of amniotic fluid. And it has nothing in its stomach that might contribute to upset.

On any long trip, especially one taken near term, a woman ought to allow for the possibility that she might require medical help somewhere. All that is needed is a list of physicians' names and addresses along the way, which her own doctor can provide.

There are all sorts of stories about women who have miscarried while off on a trip. The trip didn't cause it; they probably would have miscarried anyway, and the only reason the stories are so dramatic is that the women were out in the boondocks at the time it happened.

Late in pregnancy, it might be a different story. The mechanism that triggers labor is not at all understood, so it is easy to blame the strain of a trip if this mechanism is set off early.

But the real point is that if you go into labor while you're off traveling, you may be separated from the facilities and the people you need to help you. Therefore, any travel planned for the last eight weeks of pregnancy ought to include emergency arrangements for getting you delivered safely.

Airlines are leery of grossly pregnant women who get on their airplanes, and for good reason. They may require you to present a physician's certificate attesting that you are not likely to complicate the flight by going into labor while aloft. There's nothing in the nature of flight itself that will trigger labor, but the airlines believe, quite reasonably, that they are in the business of delivering people to destinations, not babies to their mothers.

A pregnant woman on an airplane is a lot like a furtive man carrying a bag that ticks—they both look like trouble.

The only exception that applies to air travel at any time in pregnancy is in the case of a small airplane that is not pressurized as are the commercial airliners. Oxygen gets scarce above 10,000 feet, and any pregnant woman needs a steady and dependable supply. If she's deprived of it during the first three months of pregnancy she could harm her baby. At any other time she will be the most vulnerable passenger aboard, because all pregnant women have a relative anemia that boosts their need for oxygen higher than that of people who have not had to expand blood volume to accommodate a baby.

The most important trip a woman must make, of course, is the one that takes her to the hospital.

When contractions begin in earnest, a pregnant woman faces a moment of truth. She is about to depart from home—if she's lucky enough to be there at the time that labor begins—and transport herself to a large institution known only as The Hospital.

Wouldn't it be comforting to know a little more about it?

A woman who has never been a maternity patient before can benefit greatly by visiting the place ahead of time.

She can see the admitting room and learn exactly what will happen there before she goes on to the facilities where her delivery will be managed. She can tour the labor suite and learn how she'll be attended there. She can gain considerable reassurance from seeing what a delivery room looks like, and learning about the vast array of equipment to accommodate whatever needs she may have when her baby begins his progress toward birth. Finally, she can see the nursery and *post-partum* rooms where she and her baby will be tenants for four or five days.

Most of us in the field encourage such a hospital visit and will help arrange it. I believe that the more knowledge a prospective mother has, the better will be her adaptation. Not all such lore can come from her doctor.

Yet I must allow that a tour of the hospital in which a woman is to labor and deliver can sometimes be a delusion.

A woman in her eighth month who takes her husband gaily by the hand on a sunny Sunday afternoon to go in, meet a supervisor, and jauntily march through the maternity facilities can be seriously misled. She might not hear anyone moaning in discomfort, there may be only minor activity, and the place might make the impression that it is an obstetrical Shangri-La.

This is altogether different from the experience of a woman who is in the full bloom of labor at three o'clock in the morning and who comes into the hospital to find seven other patients in the throes of serious labor. This time, probably, nobody has time to be gracious to her, she may be given a hurried enema and a quick "prep"—for preparation—while others with more pressing problems are looked after.

Such an experience can knock her for a loop—especially if she happens to be a candidate for natural or prepared childbirth who expects everything to be beautiful, calm, sweet and serene.

In the modern method of delivery that this book recommends,

conditions are not likely to be at all hectic. But any woman's hospital tour will be less than useful if she doesn't take into account that the atmosphere at the time she is in labor might not be as serene as she finds it on an introductory visit.

We've given considerable space to the mother's accommodation in the hospital; what about the baby's? Most women automatically assume that their newborn infants will be cared for by experts in an immaculate nursery, kept clean and comfortable, and only brought out for an occasional feeding by the mother if a bottle is used, or when necessary if she's breast feeding.

In most hospitals, this is pretty much the story. Newborn infants need a protected environment, a controlled atmosphere and all sorts of special equipment at hand in case of crisis. Because of their helplessness, infants also benefit from the tender and concerned attention from personnel who have chosen their work largely because they happen to love babies.

Most infants require only routine attention; they could hardly be less aware that they have access to incubators, oxygen equipment and ultraviolet lamps.

But two or three per cent of all babies will encounter some acute problems of survival, which is good enough reason to have all the apparatus present and constantly ready for use.

Some hospitals make a special effort to keep normal, healthy babies in the custody of their normal, healthy mothers. This idea is called rooming-in, and it is not so new. In the early days of hospital delivery it was standard practice for mother and baby to stay together, which they had to do if the baby was born at home.

But as more was learned about the importance of keeping babies protected from infection, the super-clean nursery was created for the isolation of babies from the germs they might encounter before they were able to marshall defenses against them. And for a long period of time, the confinement of babies to the nursery was the general rule in most American hospitals. But with our advances in control and prevention of infection, the rooming-in plan has had something of a revival.

An important motive for the change is the psychology involved.

It is the belief of rooming-in advocates that babies, small as they are, get lonely. They have a need for the cuddling and warmth of their mothers. When a hungry baby in the care of its mother begins to cry, it gets fed. But in a nursery, a baby must either get hungry on schedule or cry until it is time to be fed.

I will certainly agree that a baby benefits from the special kind of love tendered by its mother. Perhaps it can somehow sense that this person, above all others, is communicating a series of love signals not to be duplicated by anyone else.

But I seriously doubt that, at two or three days of age, a baby can distinguish between the ministrations of Mommy and those of a well-trained nurse. It is true that a mother with nothing else to do in a hospital can respond immediately to any wants of her child. But any delay in a nursery cannot be construed as neglectful, and the expertness of the care from the loving professionals there more than makes up for the lost time.

I happen to believe that a newborn infant's crying serves a definite purpose beyond signaling that its stomach may be empty or its pants full.

We know that a newborn infant's lungs are very inexperienced at the business of inhaling and exhaling air. There are thousands of tiny lung chambers that must fill and empty rapidly if the respiratory system is to operate as intended. A baby, therefore, needs breathing exercise, and crying gives it exactly that. This is not put down to justify willful neglect of an infant howling for attention. But when an infant cannot be tended to for a few minutes because of others ahead of it, there is at least the reassuring consolation of knowing that the crying serves a useful purpose.

As for the baby sensing its own loneliness, or being depressed by an impersonal, sterile atmosphere, I remain unconvinced. Most babies get to visit with their mothers several times a day, and those who don't invariably are given extra human attention and love because of the sympathy of their attendants toward their special needs.

Have you ever read stories about abandoned babies who wind up in a hospital nursery? Every nurse in the place turns on a special flow of love and concern, and the child winds up with three full shifts of adoring mothers-by-proxy.

The same is true of a baby who cannot be brought to its mother because of its own critical needs. The tenderest care in any hospital is that given to the tiny "preemies" in their incubators.

Another reason why I do not root for rooming-in is that experienced mothers don't appreciate it. Rooming-in is almost always asked for by primiparas, who always have a few stars in their eyes. Women who have been through labor and delivery before are almost unanimous in their choice; they want rest—sweet, blissful relaxation for at least a few days before tackling the chores of another motherhood.

I'm on their side. Pregnancy is a period of hard work, especially during the last few months of hauling the heavy package around. Then comes labor, which is physically debilitating, and the trauma of delivery. After a woman has been through all three, I think she deserves a vacation. This includes time to put on a frilly bed jacket and a little make-up, and a chance to look feminine as she receives the applause and appreciation of her husband and the people close to her.

It's pretty hard for a husband to visit with his wife properly if because his new infant is present, he must put on mask, cap and gown.

Rooming-in may seem modern, but "resting-in" may be a century ahead of it. Until we develop a machine that produces instant sleep and total recovery, why not let a patient postpone intensive motherhood for the four or five days of her hospital stay? Let her enjoy the fun of just being a woman who has successfully completed womanly business.

And if her baby is healthy and of good size—seven pounds or more—she ought to be able to take some of this luxury home with her. During the brief hospital stay an effort ought to be made to eliminate the two A.M.. feeding. This is for the mother's own medical benefit, for on returning home, she'll find that the necessity for this tiring job in the small hours of the night can mean the difference between her new baby being a drag or a joy.

This is as true of women who are breast feeding. They, too, can be spared one feeding a day, but a start toward that objective ought to be made while they are in the hospital.

In planning for your stay in the hospital, remember this: Although the reason for your going there is to become a mother, while you are there you will be a patient.

Make the most of it. For motherhood is a permanent condition.

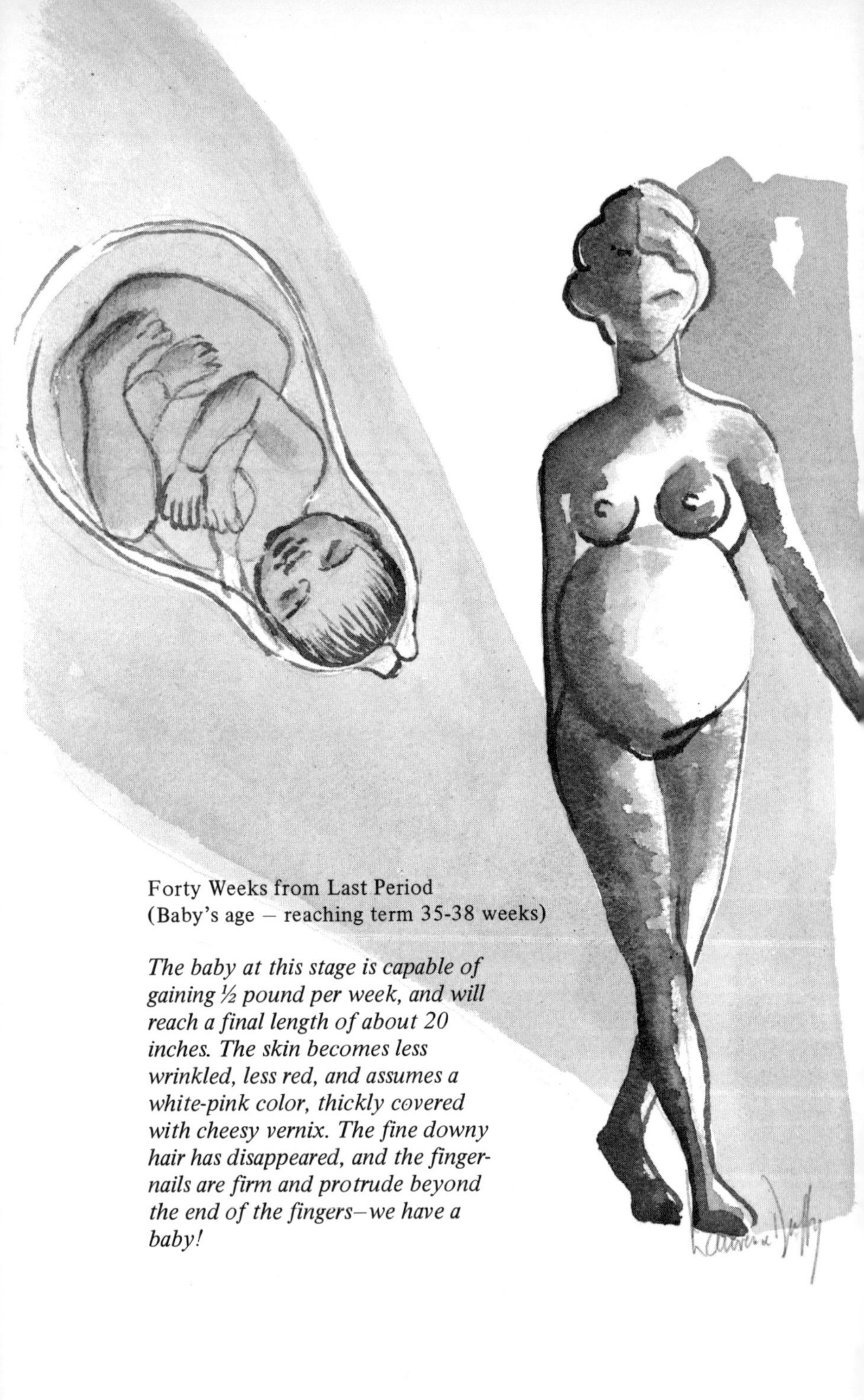

Forty Weeks from Last Period
(Baby's age — reaching term 35-38 weeks)

The baby at this stage is capable of gaining ½ pound per week, and will reach a final length of about 20 inches. The skin becomes less wrinkled, less red, and assumes a white-pink color, thickly covered with cheesy vernix. The fine downy hair has disappeared, and the finger-nails are firm and protrude beyond the end of the fingers—we have a baby!

LAST FOUR VISITS

(35th through 38th weeks)
D (delivery) minus 28 days and counting...

When will your labor begin?

That's hard to say.

Here's something to go on, however: If your menstrual cycles have been short—24 to 26 days—there is a likelihood that you will go into labor early. But if your periods always seem to have come a few days late, then your baby may also make you wait.

In the continuing growth of the baby, the last weeks are a time for finishing touches. Its weight by now is between six and seven pounds, which is very adequate to begin the process of independent life. Circulatory system, digestive tract and respiratory organs are well developed, and there is a respectable layer of fat under the skin to insure warmth.

The top of your uterus at this time may be very high—four or five finger breadths above the navel. If you have occasionally experienced sudden shortness of breath recently it is because the pregnancy is now pressing against your diaphragm, making it necessary for you to strain a little in order to fill your lungs.

Any day now, you may expect the welcome experience called "lightening." This is when the baby suddenly moves downward into the pelvis.

In a first birth, lightening can be sudden and dramatic, for the pressures surrounding the uterus tend to support the birth package until the lower segment of the uterus yields. Though the baby descends deeper into the pelvis, it does not mean that labor and delivery are necessarily imminent. In fact, the phenomenon of lightening, in a primipara, can occur two to six weeks before delivery.

In multiparous women there is usually much less of a time interval between lightening and the onset of labor; sometimes the experience is not felt at all. Labor may come directly, as the contractions of the upper portion of the uterus push the baby downward into the lower portion, which is simultaneously yielding its resistance.

Lightening, therefore, is not a reliable indicator by itself. What a woman in her final month wants to know—especially with her first baby—is how to identify labor with some assurance that labor indeed has begun.

There are three events that indicate delivery time to be at hand: the first is a change of sensation in the pelvis which may be a bit tricky for a newcomer to recognize.

Often labor begins as no more than a low backache, quite similar to the backaches frequently experienced in late pregnancy. But this pre-labor discomfort is unique, for it starts to wander.

The dull pain begins to creep around to the front. After a while you may note that your abdomen rises to a point, holds that position for a few seconds, then relaxes. You may hardly feel it at all.

Later, these risings may have a sensation to them, but they're not really painful—certainly nothing as severe as the menstrual cramps that many women have experienced in their mature lives.

Such contractions can be a reliable sign of the start of labor—but only if they are interpreted correctly.

When they become regular—by the clock on the wall, not by the clock in your head—you should measure the time intervals. At first observation they can be as far apart as once an hour. The time lapse will then shorten—30 minutes apart, 20 minutes apart.

When they are reduced to seven or eight minutes apart—by the clock on the wall, not by the clock in your head—and when they last for at least 30 seconds—then is the time to call the doctor.

But these contractions *must* be checked by a timepiece. The reason is that even the most sensible of women can get excited at the start of their first labor. If they manage to remain calm, there's a high probability that their husbands won't.

You don't believe this could happen to you? I've had women call who think they are in serious labor. "How frequent are the contractions?" I ask.

"Every minute!"

"And how long does each one last?"

"Four minutes!"

Time is relative, and seldom more so than when a primipara begins to feel the first earnest contractions telling her that the culmination of her maternal business is under way.

But the bonus of time is that there is so much of it. If you can resolve now to give the unique sensations of early labor enough time to establish a definite pattern, you are far less likely to rush to the hospital on a false alarm.

A second sign of real labor is a slight show of blood from the vagina. What's happening is that the lower segment of the uterus is beginning to retract, and the cervix is slowly dilating. Ultimately the cervix will thin out and stretch so much that it cannot be distinguished from the uterus itself. Picture a pear-shaped toy balloon; as it is inflated, the neck disappears and becomes part of the larger globe.

The reason for the slight bloody show is that the cervix, in stretching, breaks a few small blood vessels. The bleeding is usually slight, and doesn't last very long.

A third indicator is the breaking of the bag of waters. Most often this is a gush of fluid, but it can also occur as a slight dripping; the amniotic fluid may be leaking out of a small break in the envelope contained inside the uterus.

Breaking of the bag of waters, even when expected, can be a startling experience. Sometimes it may motivate a panicky dash to the telephone to deliver the message, "Doctor! I've just broken the bag of waters! What shall I do?"

We are often tempted to reply, "Move to a dry spot!" (But we don't.)

Loss of the waters is completely painless and usually poses no immediate danger. Rarely, if the baby happens to be high in the uterus, the rush of fluid can wash down the umbilical cord, which presents the threat that the baby's head can then press down on the cord, thus cutting off its blood supply.

But the doctor will be alert to this possibility from his most recent examination of the patient. If the presenting part was already low in the pelvis there will be little chance of the cord coming by. If this is so he will probably tell the woman to stay at home and wait for steady labor to begin, which it will most likely do in a short time.

The three signals of labor can occur separately, or any two together, or all three in a short time. Any one of them calls for you to exercise your best rational control, call the doctor, and be ready to head for the hospital.

Steady, measured labor will progress both in frequency and intensity. The duration of each peak will also increase. If the bag of waters breaks first, and the doctor's instructions are to wait at home, labor can be expected to begin within 24 hours and will establish the expected time pattern. Let the doctor know when contractions are seven or eight minutes apart and last for 30 seconds or more. The staining that indicates the stretching of the lower uterus and cervix is not likely to precede true labor by more than 48 hours, and usually much sooner.

There is another event that may take place, though it is no indicator of when true labor may commence. You may suddenly pass a material that looks like tissue or secretion. This is the mucous plug, the "operculum" from the cervical canal. Its passing indicates that the cervix has dilated enough to free it, but it does not necessarily mean that intensive labor is imminent.

You have time to be calm and deliberate. There is no need for a dangerous, nerve-racking dash to the hospital. All you need bring with you is the baby. You will be wholly concerned with the business of labor and delivery for the next several hours. After that your main function will be to rest and sleep. Therefore, whatever you need—nightgown, housecoat, toothbrush, nursing bra—these things can be brought to you by your husband after the baby is born.

At the start of your ninth month, chances are that the trip to the hospital is still several weeks away. There is plenty of time to plan comprehensively for those things that must be prepared for your absence.

But some women just don't.

It is perfectly understandable for a woman to regard herself as indispensable to her household. She probably is. She reserves to herself those decisions that keep the place going. But while waiting for the stirrings of labor she must grant that her baby will have first priority when labor begins.

This probably sounds like very elementary advice; but your doctor can tell you incredible stories about the things some women insist upon doing *after* labor has begun. They might keep an appointment with a hairdresser, or wash an entire kitchen floor, or jump into a car to dash to a store which is having a sale they don't want to miss.

Allow for the possibility that such irrational choices may overtake you, and get the important things done early. It may be amusing, after the fact, to hear of the nutty things a woman did after going into labor, but only if the birth went well. For yourself, resolve that you will be ready for your most important adventure; anything else can wait.

Your husband will also be alert for the coming event, and may want to be with you for as much of it as possible. If he plans to stay with you during labor and even delivery, be sure to mention this to your doctor ahead of time so there will be a clear understanding.

Some doctors will advise according to the temperament of the husband. If he's a steady, dominant kind of man, he can be of positive benefit to his wife, especially if the doctor plans to use anesthesia sparingly, or if the patient intends to attempt natural childbirth.

Many doctors, however, take a dim view of having the husband in the delivery room, unless he happens to be a person of some medical orientation. Some husbands are unable to stand by comfortably while a man they hardly know makes a two- or three-inch incision in the most private part of the wife's anatomy. They don't realize that a slight rush of blood does not mean disaster. And there is scarcely a man born, medically trained or otherwise, who can refrain from a critical appraisal of the manner in which the doctor stitches up his wife's pudendum!

In my own practice I welcome nearly all husbands to be with their wives during the entire process if they wish. This is mainly because of a new method of anesthesia—continuous epidural infusion—that keeps the woman completely comfortable throughout labor and delivery.

With the wife totally free of discomfort, there is no reason why she shouldn't be further supported by having her husband with her. The time at which labor commences, however, often determines whether or not the husband can be present. If she is laboring through the morning, he may not be able to excuse himself from his employment. Or labor may occur at a time when he must take over the responsibility of children at home.

This is one reason why it is fortunate that the time for labor to begin can now be planned. The plan is not foolproof, but it works out more often than not.

Scheduling labor is possible because the woman's readiness for delivery is usually being checked weekly by her doctor during the final month. At each visit the doctor's examination of her pelvis helps determine how ready she is—how "ripe" is the cervix in its process of stretching and thinning.

Rather than wait for labor to begin on its own—and possibly at an inconvenient hour—your doctor may judge that your progress should reach a critical point on a certain day. He will arrange for you to be admitted to the hospital on that day, where he can induce the process of labor for you.

This idea is often misunderstood. Some people conclude that the doctors only do it so they can deliver at their own convenience, rather than having to respond to a call late at night or on a day off.

But such untimely calls are no less disturbing to women and their husbands than they are to doctors.

A scheduled delivery, when possible, offers advantages to the patient, the baby and the doctor. Hospitals happen to be far better staffed in the daytime than they are at night. There are more nurses, more technicians, more specialists on hand. This means that mother and baby both benefit from maximum preparedness of the hospital.

Therefore, when a doctor can reasonably estimate, say, on a Tuesday that a woman will be ready to deliver on Friday, it makes sense to have her admitted Friday morning for elective induction of labor.

A bed will be assigned to her, she will be scheduled for preparatory treatment, and her doctor will be there as expected. All of the tension and dash-for-life atmosphere can be eliminated. At least, that's the *intent*.

Of course, a woman may still go into labor spontaneously several hours or a couple of days ahead of time. In my own practice the system of scheduling elective induction seems to work out successfully in about 75 per cent of the cases, but the women who begin spontaneous labor ahead of schedule also benefit, because there are fewer patients in labor at the odd times. Those who *are* thus receive more attention from the limited staff.

Let's say it becomes necessary for you to call to report that systematic labor has begun. You'll be interested to know what your doctor does after he tells you to get started toward the hospital:

First, he will telephone the hospital to arrange for your arrival. This assures that you will be speedily admitted and taken directly to the maternity floor. There you get your prep. The lower portion of the pubic hair will be shaved because it is easier to repair an episiotomy if there is no pubic hair to get caught in the sutures. Simple reasoning, no? You will also be given an enema to empty the lower bowel and make the pelvis roomier for the baby coming through.

You will also be asked whether you have eaten any food in the past eight hours. A recent meal or snack may rule out the use of general anesthesia, for there is a danger of vomiting, which can cause serious breathing problems in a woman not conscious enough to prevent the vomitus from blocking her airways. This is the reason for a most important instruction: When you suspect labor, don't eat *anything.* Women who are to be induced are told to fast at least from midnight on the day they are due to enter the hospital.

After the prep, you will be made comfortable in the labor room, and the doctor will be informed of your progress. Nurses make timings of your contractions and estimates of their intensity. They also monitor your baby's heartbeat by stethoscope. From its changing location they can help calculate the downward progress of the baby into the pelvic area.

In order to keep their hands free, maternity nurses wear a head stethoscope. When they want a new bearing, they bend their heads down until the stethoscope bell touches the patient's abdomen.

The doctor makes a more precise estimation of progress by his manual examination. He may do so through the rectum, but he can determine your condition much more accurately by feeling the cervix directly, through the vagina. Rectal examination is an old safety precaution, practiced in deference to what was formerly considered a danger of infection from examination of an open cervix. But new techniques make it possible to do a clean, judicious vaginal examination of the cervix early in labor.

This examination is not "aseptic," according to operating room standards—no examination of the pelvis can be. But it can be done with virtually no chance of introducing infection.

The doctor measures how open the cervix has become by the number of fingers he can insert into it. This is the key to the advance of labor. Long before the Westinghouse Company adopted its motto, obstetricians held to the precept that "progress is our most important product." How far downward has the baby moved in a measured period of time? How frequent and intense are your contractions? How much enlargement is there in the dilatation of the cervix? These are the indications of your progress toward delivery.

As the baby descends through the birth canal the mother's capacities are being tested. So are the baby's. The woman's job is to move the baby along, to deliver it to the exit. This process puts a strain on the baby. Its head and body are being rhythmically squeezed by uterine contractions, and its support from the placenta is being constantly strained by the pressure. The doctor needs to know how *both* of his patients are doing all the way. A remarkable new electronic development now makes it possible for him to monitor the intensity of the mother's efforts and their simultaneous effect on the baby.

During the first stage of labor the doctor can apply through the cervix an electrode which clips to the baby's head or buttocks—whichever is the presenting part. This electrode picks up the baby's heartbeat and produces a tracing of it on moving graph paper.

The doctor also introduces a pressure catheter which measures the intensity of the mother's contractions, tracing them on the same paper. In this way he knows at every moment how mother and baby are doing in their joint effort to complete the birth successfully. If the baby is being adversely affected by labor, or if the character of the mother's labor is not up to snuff, he will know it at once and be able to respond accordingly.

This process, however, is so new and so sophisticated that it is not generally available. But it is proving to be such a boon to the practice of obstetrics that it is bound to become widespread and available in most well-run hospitals.

And how will *you* be doing in the meantime? There are all kinds of labor rooms in America, and all sorts of women in them. You might as well be prepared.

There might be one woman present who is lost in concentration as she tries to implement her training for natural or prepared childbirth. There could be someone who reacts to a certain medication by howling like a banshee. Or you may find yourself with women who are blissfully and comfortably advancing through labor, chatting as unconcernedly as though sitting under hair dryers.

These last are likely to be beneficiaries of the modern method of anesthesia mentioned earlier—continous epidural infusion. In this method a common painkiller, similar to one used by dentists, is introduced into the tissues of the back just at the point where the main nerves of the spinal column branch out.

Instead of being put into the spinal column itself, late in labor, this anesthesia goes into the soft tissues beside the spine, and it is begun early so as to assuage all the pain of labor as well as that of delivery and repair.

Another needle is introduced into an arm vein so that medication to intensify contractions can be given if the anesthesia slows them down.

The combined effect of the two materials is to permit labor to progress normally, yet keep the patient absolutely free of pain. A labor room in which women are receiving this improved form of anesthesia is a happy place, free of anguish.

During the period of labor, your doctor may try to verify his assessment of the relationship between the size of the baby and the size of your pelvis. The match is most often favorable, but if there is doubt, he may want to see X-rays of pelvis and baby. The exposure is so slight there need be no concern of harm to either. Once your capability to deliver is assured, all that remains is for labor to continue under constant monitoring until it is apparent that delivery is imminent.

The contractions of the upper portion of the uterus are only half of the process of labor. At the same time that the powerful muscles are at work above, the lower segment of this remarkable organ is also doing its job. Slowly but steadily it is yielding, stretching, accommodating its passenger. The cervix is being taken up by this action so that it blends more and more with the uterus, and opens wider to permit passage of the baby.

This is a beautifully coordinated process; it involves the Passage, the Passenger and the Powers. The passage becomes ever more accessible. The passenger descends deeper into it. The powers of the mother, pushing from above and yielding from below, help the baby to move safely along a corridor that in the nonpregnant condition would appear impossibly inadequate.

This is the business for which your body has been making preparations. It is a nine-months-long countdown that will continue with no "holding time" until you reach the delivery room. And the entire sequence has been controlled by a bodily computer so stunningly complex that we are still in awe of its capabilities.

Ultimately we may come to understand precisely what happens to turn on the mechanism of labor, and why it proceeds at the chosen pace. At present these are mysteries involving the subtle chemistries of the body, inscrutable relationships between nerve signals and muscular response, and a battery of reserve facilities to keep all systems *go*.

Meantime, be assured that skilled human assistance is at hand, ready to intervene. All that is needed is the word from Mission Control.

DELIVERY
(AT OR ABOUT 38 WEEKS)

allow me to help you with that bundle, madam

There's a peculiar contradiction about the final days of pregnancy. Though the wait over the last few months may have seemed interminable, when labor finally does begin in earnest, many women suddenly wish they had a little more time. They wish labor was not quite so irreversible.

This is understandable. "Labor" is one of the most accurate terms in medicine; it is hard, physical work. But attitude can make it easier, especially if a woman has some tangible guide. The element of time, for example, can be fairly well bracketed.

A woman in the process of moving her first baby to the point of delivery is likely to be in labor for something between ten and thirteen hours. The largest number of primiparas will deliver between seven and nine hours after regular contractions have begun; but there is such wide variance from this norm that the average of labor time for primiparas works out to the other figure—10 to 13 hours. Obviously this results from the extremes at both ends: primiparas who negotiate labor very quickly, and those who must work many extra hours before they are ready to deliver.

For women who have delivered before—multiparas—the duration of labor will probably be shorter than required for their first babies, though not necessarily shorter than for any or all of the others. Five to seven hours applies to the majority; but again, there are enough exceptions to produce an average of eight hours.

Young women tend to have shorter labor, whether with their first babies or with others. A woman over 35 in her first pregnancy will probably labor an hour to an hour and a half longer than a younger one.

But these are no more than the loosest of guidelines, because they are entirely statistical. There are so many variables that might apply to the individual woman, that her best attitude might be one of cheerful resignation: plan for the maximum, with confidence that the doctor will be there to help if the time is extended.

There is no accurate means of predicting how much or how little your own muscular powers will help. The doctor may be able to give you a time estimate based upon the relative size of your pelvis and of the baby. A small baby, obviously, can pass through a large pelvis in a much shorter time. This fact won't change whether the woman is young, old, fat or thin.

Something you can rely on, however, is that progress will be accurately assessed repeatedly along the way. Each of the doctor's several examinations tells him how far the baby has moved in a known time period. If he is not satisfied with the rate of advance, he will take appropriate action.

A first birth, particularly, is closely watched because there is no past performance to serve as guide. The reason that the terms primipara and multipara are used as designations in maternity departments is so that everyone involved—obstetrician, anesthetist, residents and nurses— will know which set of considerations applies to each patient in the process of labor and delivery.

Any woman in labor is entitled to the assurance that priority is neither withheld nor granted according to whether she is a primipara or a multipara. The distinction is made because each status has distinctive characteristics to be accounted for in the professional techniques involved.

For a first baby, for example, a key factor is the dilatation of the cervix, which has never had to undergo this process before. This is what the doctor will check most closely as labor proceeds.

But an experienced mother's cervix has already been tested. It can be counted upon to "remember" the process. Unless the new baby is significantly larger than her others, it can be expected to come along easily as the cervix dilates.

All of these considerations apply to both spontaneous and

electively induced labor. There is a condition which changes the rules altogether: that is when a complication occurs before term is reached and the doctor must force the process of labor to begin in order to safeguard the health of mother or baby, or both.

The cause can be toxemia, diabetes, a high level of Rh antibodies, or any other urgent medical reason for separating mother and baby. If the crisis occurs between the 32nd and the 35th weeks, the woman is really not ready to be delivered, so she may not respond to attempts to start labor. If she is a primipara, most often she simply *cannot* be induced. The baby will have to be taken by caesarian section, because the untried cervix will not yield to the contractions from above. Her labor will therefore be self-canceling and useless. I believe she is committed to caesarian section for her subsequent babies, for we never can be sure that the area of the scar in the uterus will stand up under strong labor.

When labor is to be induced it is usually done by simply breaking the bag of waters with an instrument. The doctor carefully examines through the cervix to find a point within that is safely away from the baby. Here he perforates the thin envelop in which the baby is housed. There is a release of fluid, and labor can be expected to begin shortly thereafter.

In addition to this action, or instead of it, the doctor may use a drug to start contractions. This drug was originally obtained from the lobe of the pituitary gland, but it is now made synthetically. Its effect is amazingly selective. It causes the uterus to contract, yet has almost no other effect in the body. The original trade name of the medication, Pitocin, has virtually become a medical term, even when other forms are used. Pitocin can generally be counted upon to start uterine contractions which the body will then take up on its own.

Sometimes, when labor is to be forced early, the cervix is not ready. The doctor may use pitocin until the cervix dilates enough so that he can gain access to break the bag of waters. The patient might be kept on pitocin for a whole day, then allowed a night's rest. In the morning she will receive the drug again in hopes it will help to further dilate the cervix.

Now and then labor is going along nicely, then all of a sudden progress stops. Contractions may continue, but the baby does not move, or the cervix does not continue to dilate. Now the mother and the doctor face the prospect of prolonged labor and what to do about it.

The Three P's must be evaluated again: Is the Passage large enough? Is the Passenger too large? Have the Powers failed?

Modern obstetrical practice generally follows the rule that the longer the period of labor, the fewer are the options for relief. Personally, when the time reaches 14 hours, I want to know all that can be known about the reasons for delay; at 18 hours I want to make a firm decision, possibly to terminate the effort by taking the baby surgically.

The most common cause of prolonged labor is a big baby. When the baby can be shown by X-ray and palpation to be too large for the pelvis, the doctor will alter his plans ahead of time. But suppose there is a degree of doubt? Measurements may show, for example, that the size of the baby's head and the size of the pelvis are about the same. Can it be assumed that the pelvis will yield? Making such measurements precisely is quite difficult. Some current investigators believe they have developed a method by which compatibility between baby and pelvis can be quite accurately determined—at least enough to direct a decision for caesarian section more confidently than has been possible in the past. This method will certainly bear fruit after it accumulates more applications. Meantime, it remains difficult to estimate the adaptability of passenger to passage. When the measurements are close, favoring the passage slightly, we usually let the woman attempt delivery. But she must show progress.

As labor continues beyond 14 hours, several unhappy conditions intensify: The mother begins to tire, so her contractions become less effective. She may become dehydrated. The supply of oxygen that she can transmit to her baby begins to diminish. And her reaction to pain may begin to frustrate the entire effort.

Fortunately, obstetrical surgery has now become a dependable alternative.

Whether the length of labor be normal or otherwise, the intensity of pain is a prime medical consideration. Pain serves no purpose if it stifles the function that causes it. This is the main reason for analgesia, which is medication to lessen pain, and for anesthesia, which is to prevent pain altogether.

The process of delivering a baby can never be guaranteed to be free of discomfort and pain. With the fullest possible regard for the school of natural or prepared childbirth, it must be admitted that the method is not successful for everyone who tries it.

Most obstetricians accept as a fact that labor will be painful, and take to themselves the responsibility for keeping the patient as comfortable as possible. This is probably why so many of us tend to be a bit wary of the first-time mother who comes sailing into the hospital, smiling in spite of her twinges, and insists that she won't even look at an aspirin while Nature is at work.

If we happen to know from examination that she has a big baby and a small pelvis, her optimism is not convincing. This is why any woman who wishes to attempt one of the allegedly painless methods should find out well ahead of time how her doctor feels about it. She also ought to be ready to accept his advice if a condition arises that causes a level of pain totally unrelated to her preparation for unmedicated delivery.

It is no more of a disgrace for a woman to experience difficulty despite her hopes and training than it is for a fine figure skater to stumble over a bobby pin on the ice. Unfortunately the natural and prepared methods often engender a high degree of zeal and fervor among women who try them, and they tend to punish themselves for the innocent response of feeling pain they were told would not arise. If such women are told during pregnancy to take iron pills, they will take them; an iron deficiency has nothing to do with one's attitude toward having a baby. By the same reasoning they ought to be willing to accept medication and anesthesia to assuage pain when the doctor clearly sees that they need it, just as they needed the iron pills.

The main avenue of research for such pain relief in obstetrics has been toward finding drugs that reduce discomfort in the mother without adversely affecting the baby.

In the days of what was called "twilight sleep," a combination of morphine and scopolamine was used. This put the mother out of the picture effectively, but it caused serious problems of respiration in the baby because it was literally born "doped up."

Over the years, other drugs such as demerol and leritine—intended as substitutes for morphine—have been tried, but they too get into the baby's system, and, if used in large amounts, which are sometimes necessary to comfort the mother effectively, result in problems for the infant.

Scopolamine by itself has an amnesic effect; it does not significantly reduce pain during labor and delivery, but it tends to help the patient forget the torturous episode when it's over. Women on this drug are terribly hard to control during labor; they tend to thrash around, scream, and generally cause an awful rumpus on the maternity floor. They can be even more difficult on the delivery table, and must be put to sleep for the actual birth. Scopolamine patients tire themselves out and may become disoriented to the point that they are of no help when asked to bear down.

There are several inhalation anesthesias in use, but the main point about all of them is that they must be mixed with plenty of oxygen so that they will not depress the baby's ability to breathe after it is born.

In modern anesthesiology, gases that produce sleep are almost never given in high concentration as they once were. A generous level of oxygen must be included, for the child remains utterly dependent upon oxygen through the umbilical cord, and must carry a reserve of oxygen-enriched blood to sustain it until it gains access to the outside air and can begin its own process of respiration. In effect, then, the comfort of the mother must be measured against the security of the child. Sometimes, in balancing this equation, the deficit must be paid in discomfort and pain.

Childbirth pain usually becomes most intense near the moment of delivery; this is also the time when the doctor will do the episiotomy— cutting of the tissues to prevent their tearing, and to provide a wider opening. Inhalation anesthesia is usually given just prior to both of these events.

Without episiotomy the tissues will tear anyway. It has been found that a neat surgical incision, properly repaired, heals better and sooner than does the irregular laceration that is almost inevitable without the operation.

In natural and prepared childbirth, doctors also use episiotomy, though they may do so without anesthesia. One medical advocate of the unmedicated method says the mother does not feel the pain of the tearing or of a surgical incision. I don't believe it. But even if she is able to endure that moment, the repair of the incision or laceration is something else again. A sharp needle and suturing material must be passed repeatedly through extremely sensitive tissues over a period of several minutes. The woman must have some kind of anesthetic, usually local, for this to be done.

With inhalation anesthesia, both episiotomy and delivery take place with the patient unconscious. This fact has become a major complaint against the use of gas, because the woman misses the most impressive part of the episode. She does not know when her baby is born or how quickly it started to breathe, or how it looks. In fact, she doesn't know anything at all, until she regains consciousness.

For this reason, an alternate method of pain control has been more popular in recent years. It is called conduction anesthesia, introduced into the spinal column. Most women know it as "saddle block."

In this method the pain-controlling material is injected into the spinal column when it becomes apparent that the woman is about to deliver. The intent of saddle block is to anesthetize the body from the pelvic area down, so that the uterine contractions are not stifled, yet the woman will not feel their pain.

Such a spinal anesthesia is used not only so that the woman can be aware of the birth sequence; it is always preferred when she is known to have food in her stomach.

The big advantage of continous epidural infusion, the pain-control method that I favor and have already described, is that it can be used for hours—in fact, for the entire period of labor and delivery. In cases where caesarian section has proved necessary, epidural infusion has been continued in the operating room, where it has also served well.

The anesthesia used in epidural, combined with pitocin as necessary to maintain the intensity of uterine contractions, may add an hour or so to the duration of labor. But the bonus to both mother and child is enormous. The mother is fully conscious throughout her labor, she is completely free of pain and totally alert. Because she is altogether unmedicated, she can watch the delivery process in a mirror above the table. She will hear her baby's first cries, which may occur spontaneously before its entire body is out of the birth canal.

There is none of the wooziness that follows inhalation anesthesia, and none of the headache that can follow a spinal. During delivery of the placenta and repair of the episiotomy, the mother can look at her new baby in the incubator, which is usually moved into her visual range. Because she remains fully conscious, she and her husband can review the entire affair together, which is an especially joyful experience. If for any reason the husband missed actually seeing the delivery, at least his wife can give him a vivid account of what happened.

And what about the baby? In its first moments of life it can howl lustily, since such excellent breathing exercise is uninhibited by medication. This helps inflate its lungs and stimulate circulation so that the wiggling and flexing of arms and legs can be tried out in the open for the first time.

As with nearly every major advance in medicine, epidural anesthesia has possible disadvantages. Since the uterus is not as relaxed, full anesthesia may have to be used when it is necessary to manipulate the baby, as in breech presentation. (The same is required in saddle block.)

But this is a matter the doctor can cope with. Part of his responsibility is to develop the skill to manipulate a baby who is in an unfortunate position, or to remove a placenta that does not come along easily. Also, there are cases in which the anesthesia simply doesn't work. The needle can be properly placed, the material injected as usual, but for reasons that defy explanation, pain continues, and some other means must be employed.

Another disadvantage is that if something abnormal occurs, the mother will probably be aware of it. She is totally conscious and intensely interested in what is happening. If her baby does not breathe and cry immediately, she knows it. If it is not physically perfect, an attempt may be made to hide this fact, and most often she can conclude why. Suddenly the delivery room becomes quiet. Nurse, anesthetist and obstetrician, who may have been chatting amiably a moment before, become hushed. The patient instantly picks up the tension. What had been a moment before a scene of excitement and wonder becomes a place of concern and sorrow.

But who is to say that bad news can ever be broken easily? It is no less painful for a woman to accept the news of a lost or marred baby hours later than when it is first known.

That is why this slim possibility does not dim my enthusiasm for epidural anesthesia. It is a magnificent way to have babies, providing the benefits of unmedicated childbirth without the pain. No analgesia need be used at any time during labor. There is no problem if the husband wishes to be present for both labor and delivery. Best of all, his wife knows that she will be a thoroughly presentable female throughout.

As usual in any newly-formed idea, the one who first promulgates it sometimes tends to overdo and can give the entire movement an unsavory aura. For example, Grantly Dick-Read, in *Childbirth Without Fear*. Dick-Read, although an avowed hypnotist and a mystic whose techniques really worked only for him, forced the medical profession to give less medication to women in labor. This is one of the great advances in obstetrics, and although I disagreed and still do with Dick-Read's approach, I am in awe of his ability to have turned us around on overmedication. Millions of women have benefited from this otherwise misguided *accoucheur*.

So with LeBoyer. He has focused our attention on the baby as an individual, one to be considered before, during, and after delivery as an entity apart from its mother. He and I disagree on some issues, such as why a baby cries after delivery. He believes it is from the pain of delivery, the shock of meeting the new hostile world. I believe that a baby cries out of the need to expand its lungs, to start breathing so that life can be maintained. Nevertheless, LeBoyer, also a man of mystical bent, has contributed greatly to our understanding of the newborn as an individual, with the rights and perquisites of a person.

At long last now we can talk about your baby as a living individual. For with delivery he—or she—suddenly becomes a human person, howling for attention. Just as suddenly the baby becomes a patient of doctor and hospital. So how is it treated?

Quite respectfully. For a starter, babies are seldom held upside down and spanked on the bottom to make them breathe these days. Usually they start breathing spontaneously, because medications that formerly inhibited the process are now used so sparingly.

If there should be a slight delay in the start of respiration, the doctor may tap the bottom of the baby's feet or give a slight slap on the rump. There may be a soft mucous plug in the baby's pharynx, which the doctor will remove with a suction bulb.

Next, the umbilical cord will be doubly clamped off an inch or so away from the baby's abdomen. The cord is then cut between the clamps, and the baby is passed to the nurse. She takes it in a towel, cleans it up a bit, and puts it into the incubator. There, its first few minutes will be spent in crying, moving about, and in general adapting itself to the new world around it.

It is a delightful sight for the mother to watch, which is what she usually does. There is still much to be done for her—delivering the placenta, stitching the episiotomy—I haven't seen a mother yet who hasn't preferred to crane her neck a little so she can watch the fascinating show going on inside the incubator.

Very early in this sequence the baby will be tagged with a bracelet that is the mate to one worn by the mother, which came into the delivery room with her. No other baby in the hospital or in the world can get that tag. The worry over getting the wrong baby bedevils every mother, so make it a point to watch for the installation of the proper tag during the period right after delivery.

The baby's eyes will be washed out, as is required by law in most states. A mild solution of silver nitrate is generally used. Many states are changing to a penicillin solution to obviate the remote danger that the silver nitrate might be improperly mixed. In either case the purpose is to prevent infection of the baby's eyes by venereal disease that might be present in the mother's birth canal.

In cases of Rh involvement, blood samples are taken from the umbilical cord and from the mother to determine whether a transfer of Rh antibodies may have taken place.

The child will then be seen by the pediatrician, before or after being taken to the nursery. It is an absolute axiom that the best care given in any hospital by anybody is given to the babies in the nursery.

And what about you, there on the delivery table? You may develop a few qualms, unless you know something about delivery—especially if you are awake and alert while it's going on.

It is important to understand that there is a significant difference between bleeding and hemorrhage. There will be some bleeding from the incision of episiotomy, but it will be quickly controlled. There will also be a moderate flow of blood during and after delivery. None of this need disturb you; the only alarming thing about blood is its color, which tends to make a little look like a lot.

If there should happen to be bleeding beyond what is normal, it will be obvious immediately to the medical team around you, and they will know how to take care of it.

Lost blood can be replaced. This is why most hospitals request patients to have someone in their families make a donation to a blood bank ahead of time. Despite such blood programs, however, most doctors would be a lot happier if more standby blood were readily available. Obstetrical surgery will be vastly improved when the same standard of immediate blood availability demanded for other surgery applies.

Remember that although you are a hospital patient at the time of your delivery, you are most likely not a *sick* patient. You are a healthy woman who is engaged in a normal process. If you lose more blood than is expected, you will be in good shape again immediately when the lost blood is replaced.

Few women require service and assistance beyond that which is supplied in a routine delivery. Hardly any of them expect this, so when it happens, they become alarmed. But as is true with any new experience, you can always manage better if you know something about what to expect.

For instance, it may be necessary to use forceps to assist in the delivery. Immediately, the mother begins to worry that this instrument will mar the baby. Not true. Modern forceps are beautifully designed to help, not hurt, the baby.

Forceps are almost never used until the baby's head is low in the pelvis and has passed through the cervix. They are carefully fitted, one part at a time, with the doctor using his hand to protect the side of the baby's head as each part is applied.

Then the two parts are joined at the fulcrum, and the doctor makes a gentle downward and upward motion to guide the baby's head past the symphysis bone at the center of the mother's pelvis. When the head emerges, the forceps are removed, and the delivery is completed by a combination of the mother's own power and the doctor's manual guidance.

Low forceps are generally used if the patient is under spinal or epidural anesthesia, or if an inhalation anesthesia is necessary before her own labor has pushed the baby's head far enough for the doctor to receive it. They are always used with great care; a primary skill of obstetrics is the use of forceps and hands to expedite delivery. It is one of the things your doctor does best, therefore, one that need concern you least.

Another special skill that may be called for is delivering a baby that is not presented head downward in the usual vertex position—the breech.

In a breech delivery, the doctor can usually guide the baby's legs and body through the narrow portion of the birth canal. As the baby's lower body emerges, the doctor takes it along his forearm. It is important to have the baby covered with a towel for warmth so that it will not gasp in response to the comparative cold of the delivery room. In an attempt to breathe before the head is free of the mother, the baby could take in fluid that might cause it to cough or choke.

The major concern in a breech delivery is that the head, which is the largest part of the baby's body, doesn't arrive until last, so its adaptability to the pelvis is not altogether known until then. But nearly always it can be gently manipulated through the passage without real difficulty. Babies are amazingly adaptable to this passage whether they come frontwards or backwards.

The most common difficulty encountered in breech delivery is that progress slows or stops altogether. Continuous advance through the birth canal is always important, but it is decisive in breech presentation. So long as there is progress, the doctor can manage the manipulation necessary to deliver. But when progress stops before the baby becomes accessible, it usually means the woman must be moved into the operating room and the baby taken by caesarian section.

There is one school of thought that says all primiparous breeches should be sectioned out of hand. I don't believe this. But if a breech doesn't continue to make good and regular progress, that is, both descent and dilatation—if there is any holdup or interruption in the orderly process of labor—the woman becomes a good candidate for section.

When delivery from below must be ruled out, whether ahead of time because of disease or complication, or at the last minute due to difficulty in the labor or delivery room, there is a support facility nearby.

Close to the delivery room there is an operating room that is kept completely prepared. It has sterile instruments, gowns, and full anesthetic facilities. When surgical delivery of a baby becomes necessary, it can be done without delay.

This is caesarian section, which has become a routine procedure. Though the operation is centuries old, it is only within the past 25 years or so that the major dangers have been removed from it. If Julius Caesar was indeed born this way, as the legend claims, it is certain that his mother died as a result.

For hundreds of years, caesarian section remained a desperate measure resorted to in the hope of saving a baby whose mother was lost. But with the development of germ-free surgical technique, the perfection of anesthesia, the discovery of antibiotics, and most especially, the ability to replace lost blood, the major hazards were removed. Caesarian section has now become the benevolent bail-out for a mother and baby in trouble.

It is also a much simpler and safer operation. The incision is now made across the lower section of the uterus, from which the baby can very speedily be removed. Repair and healing are much more dependable in this area, also. In fact, some obstetricians feel that if there is no compelling reason for caesarian in a subsequent pregnancy, the patient may be allowed to deliver from below.

I disagree. And I would say that the majority of obstetricians favors the dictum: "once a section, always a section." The scar across a uterus that has been sectioned is strong, but the area around the scar may not be. If a perforation should occur from the strain of a subsequent delivery effort, the complications can be horrendous. We will surely lose the baby, we will probably lose the uterus, and in extreme instances, we may lose the mother.

But since most women can have as many babies as they want by caesarian, it makes sense to use the safer method.

Of course there is a certain psychological satisfaction for a woman to deliver from below by the normal physiological process. If she has all of her babies by section she may feel unfulfilled. But I would much rather try to persuade her that she proves her sense of motherhood better by being cautious than she does when she takes the chance that she might leave her children motherless. The risk of letting a once-sectioned woman deliver may run that high.

The prospect of repeated caesarian sections need be no handicap.

Some women have had large families, undergoing surgery every time. There is one I know of who probably holds the all-time indoor-outdoor track record: 12 caesarian deliveries.

Whether your baby is delivered by surgery or from below, there is the promise of a great experience when it is over. For you will be able to lift your head from your pillow in the hospital bed, look down the length of your body, and see for yourself that the mountain is gone.

You will be FLAT, my dear, and it's a nice condition to be in.

POST-DELIVERY

days in the life of her highness

After the delivery is over, most women entertain a fairly understandable desire: they'd like to have a meeting, however brief, with the man who served as co-sponsor for this major event.

If the woman has had general anesthesia, the meeting may have to be deferred. If not, she isn't likely to remember much of it. She will be only fuzzily conscious, she may be slightly nauseous, and she may still feel the effects of medication during labor.

Patients who have had spinal anesthesia are somewhat handicapped by the fact that they must lie still with head absolutely flat in order to fend off the severe headache that may result from undue motion of the head before the spinal fluid has regained its normal balance.

Women who have been successful at delivering without medication or anesthesia may feel a bit fatigued, though emotionally elated. However, they are usually delighted to visit with their husbands shortly after delivery.

The same is true of patients who have had epidural. Nearly always they are able to see their husbands with no fear of displaying signs of distress or debilitation. But in hospitals that do not provide for the presence of the husband at delivery, the visit of wife and husband must defer to the visit of husband and doctor. It is an unwritten rule that nobody talks to the husband until the doctor officially brings the news. This is a responsibility that we obstetricians regard as a privilege, for it is almost always an experience of pleasure and amusement.

It's fun to breeze into the waiting room and say something along these lines: "I've got a baby boy to give away—any takers?"

Nearly always the husband's first question is, "How is my wife?" When he is told that she is fine and that their baby is busy at the management of independent life, the sex of the child hardly ever seems to make any real difference. It doesn't seem to matter if a man has been harping for nine months about fathering a daughter, or if his fingers have been crossed against the possibility of a seventh consecutive son; in that moment he is invariably pleased by whatever the doctor tells him.

This reaction is so constant that it makes a good argument against research efforts to identify or control the sex of a child before birth.

There are intensely enjoyable moments associated with childbirth; to be with a mother following the successful delivery of a healthy child is one of them. To bring the news to a proud and delighted father is another. A third and special pleasure is to bring husband and wife together with their new child as soon as possible after the event. I regard it as an important objective of the obstetrician to preserve and enhance these meaningful moments.

The ideal is for the husband to be able to see his wife while the full joy of successful childbirth is upon her. He can touch her, and kiss her, and hear her tell how she watched the entire birth in a mirror.

The new baby will also be there in its incubator, so that husband and wife can look at it together. Such a meeting has an enormous bonding power for any family; for if childbirth is a beautiful experience, it becomes all the more so from being shared without the distractions of discomfort, disorientation and undue delay.

Our new approaches to anesthesia make this more frequently possible. Today we even allow the husband to be in the room to sit at the head of the operating table with his wife while Caesarian section is being done. This is a really new concept (at least at this revision of this book) and helps to give the same sense of fulfiliment that parents get from a delivery that is conducted vaginally. However, actually watching the section through a mirror may be somewhat unsettling for both husband and wife, so this is not yet part of the New Deal.

As facilities and personnel for newer techniques in anesthesia become more generally available, it is entirely possible that the gap between patient and doctor regarding the woman's attitude toward the importance of her own contribution to the effort will narrow. Most obstetricians would encourage a woman who wants to deliver while fully alert if she would be willing to accept help should her own efforts at pain control prove inadequate.

The objection of obstetricians to current attitudes of natural and prepared childbirth trainees is that some of them seem more anxious to be able to say, "I won," than: "We have a child." On the face of the evidence of results, it would seem that epidural infusion is the perfect complement to the non-medicated method should difficulty arise.

Sometimes such difficulty prevents the immediate reunion of husband and wife. If she has lost an unusual amount of blood, the husband must wait until she responds to transfusion. Caesarian section may keep the couple apart until the mother is capable of a meaningful visit. If the baby has been lost, or has been born with some tragic abnormality, the meeting between husband and wife will be one surrounded by tragedy.

Yet even in such an instance, the woman will be in the presence of the one person best able to offer support, comfort and love.

In this connection, I must say a special word about Catholic patients and Catholic obstetricians. I know a great many Catholic men in this profession, and I can think of none who would elect, upon religious grounds, to save a baby at the cost of a mother's life. Yet I receive patients, as I know other non-Catholic obstetricians do, who choose us for that reason alone. Often the husband will actually say, straight out, "We are Catholic, but I am bringing my wife to you because I know you won't let her die in order to save the baby."

This belief is quite unfair to Catholic obstetricians. They are equally concerned with the health and survival of both mother and child.

Furthermore, I would be very hard put to find a medical situation in which such an awful choice need be made. A Catholic physician, like any other, is concerned with two objectives for his patients: freedom from suffering, and survival. Toward these ends he, like any doctor, grants equal consideration for mother and child.

The notion about this legendary "choice" probably arose in the days before the development of anesthesia and blood replacement, when any surgical procedure was likely to be fatal to the mother. Since death of the mother was often inevitable in such cases, physicians took those steps necessary to secure a live baby. But they were not making a choice between mother and child, for with the mother doomed, they had none.

In current obstetrical practice there is no such concern. If a woman has reasons to select a Catholic obstetrician, she need have no fear about his religious convictions affecting her and her baby.

Safety of mother and child is seldom in jeopardy during childbirth. Delivery occurs uneventfully better than 95 per cent of the time. Assuming yourself to be a member of the happy, normal majority, your next logical thought is to wonder how you are going to feel when delivery is over.

That all depends on how things go. A woman who has been a smashing success at controlling her pain without medication will feel satisfied, fulfilled and justifiably proud of herself. The patient who has been protected from pain by conduction anesthesia will also feel rather wonderful.

Those who have had medication plus general anesthesia must necessarily cope with the side effects that delay the return of a feeling of well-being.

Aside from this, however, *post-partum* patients usually feel pretty good. They are tired and quite willing to sleep, of course. But within six or seven hours of delivery, they will usually be told to sit up in bed, dangle their feet over the side, then take a few steps around the room.

This moderate exercise is extremely important; it helps to get the blood circulating better and tends to overcome the danger of blood clots forming in the legs and in the large veins of the pelvis.

In earlier days, a woman who had delivered was generally confined to bed for a week or more, as though she were dreadfully fragile. This inactivity often led to thrombophlebitis, the medical term for inflammation of the veins that can lead to clots which form in the swollen veins, then break away to move through the circulatory system.

A woman should not expect this early exercise to be a jaunty stroll down the corridor to peek in at the nursery window. She just won't be up to it. As medication and anesthesia wear off, she will find herself in a fair degree of discomfort. The early ambulation may have to be "encouraged," which is a rank euphemism. The maternity ward nurse may practically blast you out of bed, when your every inclination is to stay there. But the relentless order to get moving is for your own protection, so you might as well get up and get it over with.

A major source of discomfort is the site of the episiotomy. Remember that a fairly long incision—two or three inches—has been made and repaired in a very tender area. Several stitches have been put there, and they tend to dry and harden a little with the passage of time. So the area can feel quite sore. To ease the soreness, *post-partum* patients usually receive mild medication for three days, sometimes four. There are several choices—I use a combination of aspirin and codeine— but their purpose is simply to minimize discomfort.

There is also the phenomenon of after-pain to contend with. What happens is that the uterus endeavors to return to its normal size. It does so through contractions that are quite similar to those of labor, though much milder.

After-pains are generally stronger in multiparas, but there is no guarantee that they will not be uncomfortably felt after a first baby. But the medications are effective, and the intensity of the after-pains will diminish a bit each day.

Women who nurse their babies will feel the uterine contractions quite directly. As the baby suckles, a reaction takes place so that the uterus seems to contract in proportion to the intensity with which the baby nurses. The response is so pronounced that nursing mothers are frequently amazed by it; it is as though the baby is performing a service for its mother in return for its food. Advocates of breast feeding cite this uterine response as evidence that a woman is not only intended to nurse, but she will be better off if she does.

Many obstetricians feel that nursing merely speeds up the pace at which the uterus returns to normal size, and that there is no particular reason to hurry. Also, both nursing and non-nursing mothers usually receive ergotrate on their first day; this drug markedly accelerates the contracting of the uterus.

But it would be unfair to dismiss breast feeding with the off-handed comment that a drug makes it unnecessary. To some women breast feeding is an integral part of the birth process; they genuinely feel that their maternal experience is incomplete without it. Such women ought to nurse if they can, and obstetricians ought to encourage them.

That doesn't mean that a woman ought to be talked into breast feeding if she feels a degree of reluctance about it. Neither should nursing suddenly be decided upon by whim when she's sitting up in bed after delivery wearing a new nightgown. The decision to breast feed is one to be made long before delivery, and what's more, it ought to be trained for. If a woman has not toughened herself up by daily scrubbing for months, the pain can be severe. The baby can cause such acute discomfort and soreness as to prevent nursing altogether.

A nursing mother must also prepare herself for a certain degree of frustration, for the fact is that newborn babies don't have the faintest idea of what to do when brought to the breast. They must be guided, cajoled, persuaded and even shaken. It has been facetiously said that breast feeding is a failure until the baby gets the hang of it. And if you find that to be gross, you may be one of those women who shouldn't try it anyway.

Nature has conveniently provided a trial period for nursing. A mother's milk does not come into her breasts in quantity until the third day. Therefore, bringing the infant to its mother until then is little more than a training session. While learning, the baby may manage to swallow some of the sticky, colorless fluid exuded by the breasts at this time. This material is called colostrum; in humans it is only beneficial in helping the child learn to swallow and in serving as a mild cathartic.

It is debatable whether immunizing antibodies are given to an infant by way of the colostrum. We know that in cattle, the cow's immunities cannot pass to the calf while in the uterus, so it is extremely important that a calf nurse soon after birth for protection against disease.

But this is not true in humans. The child is born well protected by the immunities of its mother. Ingestion of colostrum may fortify this immunity to a degree, but modern obstetrical opinion believes it to be unnecessary.

Another reason for breast feeding that is often cited is its psychological effect on the baby. The child is cuddled, held close to the warmth of the mother, and is comforted by the nearness of the mother's heartbeat, which was its constant reassurance while in the womb. The flow of milk is satisfying and pleasing; its composition. of course, is close to perfection.

Yet all of this is also true of bottle feeding. The modern milk formula, dispensed from a bottle, nourishes a child just as adequately as natural milk. If the child is held close it feels its mother's warmth and feels the beat of her heart.

I would like to encourage any woman who has a strong determination to nurse her baby. If she prepares herself for it, and adapts herself and her baby to it, she can only be admired.

But the woman who cannot nurse, or who prefers not to nurse, or who is prevented from nursing by other circumstances, should not feel the slightest bit guilty about it. She is not neglecting her child, nor depriving it of an important relationship. She certainly cannot be accused of loving it less.

For the fact is that women who are able to breast feed their babies in our society are rather lucky and quite rare. They are the ones who do not have to return to a job, or who don't have several other small children deserving of attention, or husbands unsympathetic to the project.

There's a very tired joke in obstetrics on the advantages of breast feeding which, I will boldly declare, has never before been put into print by a physician: "Mother's milk is dandy because it's up off the floor where the cat can't get at it, it can be taken to movies and picnics, and it comes in such lovely containers."

The reference to the sex appeal of female breasts is not superficial; to be realistic, we must recognize that a woman's bosom is an extremely important focal point of her sexual apparatus. If a wife has the slightest intimation that her husband is disturbed by her nursing, she should take it carefully into account and decide whether pleasing him is as important as fulfilling her own maternal desires.

Some men enjoy the idea of having a wife nurse. Others are annoyed, repelled or actually made jealous by it. Since it doesn't make the slightest difference to the baby, I would recommend that the woman decide in favor of her man. After all, it was her femininity that attracted his attention in the first place, and if that femininity is not implicit in the bustline, then dedicated girl-watchers have been wasting their time for centuries.

Consider it this way: breast feeding has a dual approach. But there are also a couple of arguments against it—both well rounded!

A woman who wants to nurse will find, in most cases, that she'll be ready for it when the time comes, even if she's had a difficult delivery. Blood loss will have been replaced, she'll have had plenty of time to rest, and the baby will probably not nurse long enough, the first few times, to tire her out or make her nipples sore. While waiting for the milk to come in, the baby will receive glucose and water by bottle in the nursery. Delivery by caesarian section in no way precludes nursing.

There's another consideration to be made about breast feeding which has come to light as a result of our concern over air and water pollution. Because of widespread and perhaps indiscriminate use of insecticides, it has been shown that there is a higher content of DDT in mother's milk than is tolerated under the law in dairy milk.

The congressman who made the revelation pointed out that mother's milk would never be allowed to cross a state border, if it weren't housed in such un-invadable containers.

Whether breast or bottle is used, a woman must learn how to feed and care for her baby. Many hospitals provide classes conducted by nurses to show mothers how to encourage a reluctant eater, how to hold and lift a seemingly fragile infant, and the fairly tricky business of changing and bathing a very small child.

The babies themselves learn by experience and self-teaching. An infant on the breast finds out that, by shaking its head back and forth on contact with the breast, it can quickly locate the nipple, which it will then clamp down upon earnestly.

Most women find it convenient and comfortable to switch the baby from one breast to the other partway through the feeding. But be sure to wait until the baby eases up momentarily, for it can be very painful to try interrupting a baby who is sucking hard and getting a good flow. The reason it is wise to shift when possible is that an unused breast will later become engorged with milk. This can become so uncomfortable that the breast may have to be pumped out manually before the next feeding.

The only way to determine how much milk a breast-fed baby has taken at a given feeding is to weigh the baby before and after, which isn't too practical. But the amount of milk consumed is not usually crucial anyway. If the baby has had enough, it will be content; if not it will howl. Breast feeding will generally tire a baby more frequently and therefore will take longer than bottle feeding.

If you have twins or more, breast feeding is quite impractical. Two children cannot be nursed at once, and neither will usually get enough. This means supplementary bottles and making choices about who gets which, and that quickly becomes a nuisance.

One unarguable advantage of bottle feeding is that every now and then someone else can do it. By contrast, a nursing mother can seldom hope for more than four to eight hours of freedom from her feeding assignment. The lactation process won't let her go much beyond that without resorting to the breast pump.

I have found that one of the best measures toward speedy recuperation of the mother is the elimination of the two A.M. feeding. Both mother and baby can be trained for this while they are still in the hospital, nursing mothers included.

It may be a cry in the wilderness, but there is hardly a service more appreciated by a woman than for her husband to take the late feeding when necessary. There is a special form of agony for a woman who has tended a baby all day to have to shake herself out of sleep, change her baby, and sit through what seems positively to be the longest and slowest sequence of feed-and-burp of the day. A Legion of Maternal Honor badge should be awarded to husbands who take on this chore. You might tactfully suggest this by pointing out that hospitals regard the mother's sleep as so important that they do not bring in the babies for the late, late show.

A woman's time in the hospital has been consistently reduced over recent years. Early ambulation has helped her to recover faster, and advances in diet, asepsis and blood replacement have made it possible to shorten the ordinary stay from ten days to five days. Many hospitals are now releasing *post-partum* women after four days. But with the rising cost of hospitalization those women with a poor insurance policy or none at all may choose to leave even earlier than that. Under normal circumstances there have been no dire results from this.

During her stay the mother will be quite pleasantly occupied. She can sleep, which is often the prime luxury. She will learn how to handle her baby, who will be delightful company each time it is brought in. Discomfort will decrease steadily, and she will generally find herself more and more eager for a chance to stroll around.

Weight loss is usually dramatic. The immediate loss, comprised of baby, afterbirth and fluids, may be between 12 and 14 pounds.

The reduction continues in the hospital and at home for about two weeks, for a total of 17 or 18 pounds. If at that time she is heavier than when she began the pregnancy, the remaining pounds must be taken off the hard way—by diet and exercise.

During the hospital stay, visitors will probably be restricted to the husband, the child's grandparents, and perhaps some immediate family. Excessive visitation can be tiring to a *post-partum* patient, and since her stay in the hospital is now so short, its main purpose should be rest and recovery.

On the third hospital day we can quite confidently expect to see symptoms of *post-partum* depression, a medical condition much better known as the "baby blues." This is a combination of fatigue from labor and delivery, mild discomfort from contractions and stitches, and general loneliness. Treatment is simple—maybe a pep talk by the doctor, a thoughtful gesture by the husband, or a happy time with the baby. Sometimes all that is needed is that the woman know ahead of time that she may feel a little down, and so should try to snap herself out of it. Once in a while—very rarely—she may be given a mild perk-up drug.

The hospital diet will be generous and nutritious, with no special restrictions unless the mother is nursing. The nursing diet eliminates chocolate and any vegetables that have a cathartic action. At home nursing mothers should avoid alcohol, as this, too, will get through to the baby from the milk.

Except for mild ambulation to improve blood flow, a woman need not think about other exercise while she is in the hospital, or, for that matter, until after her six-weeks *post-partum* checkup. Until then she ought to let her body take its own time in returning organs and muscles to their natural state.

Bowel and bladder care will be just about the same as before pregnancy, except that the patient will be a little tender at the episiotomy site. Mild laxatives may be necessary to prevent straining, and she will be instructed to use soap and water after each movement to keep the stitched area clean.

There will be a bloody vaginal discharge, called lochia, that continues after delivery. For the first three or four days this will be bright red, then it becomes paler and more pinkish. After about ten days the discharge turns yellowish in color, but is mixed with a little blood. This is a product of the continuing discharge from the uterus; it has nothing to do with menstruation. You will be instructed and assisted in its care while in the hospital. At home it is easily tended to by light douches, baths and spongings. Internal sanitary devices should not be worn during this period.

There is no restriction on baths or showers. Chances are you will want to take regular sitz baths for comfort around the episiotomy. Water does not enter the vagina during these baths, so there is almost no danger of infection.

Altogether, the days in the hospital should be restful, blissful and easy to take. My apologies that advances in modern medicine have reduced the length of the vacation you so conspicuously have earned.

GOING HOME

back to the old ironing board

A stay in the hospital of five days, or four days, as is the trend, is not a very long time for a woman who has made such a major effort as is demanded in the delivery of a child.

Strangely, most women find it long enough. They enjoy the luxury of bed rest, the novelty of visiting with the new baby, and the special attentions of husband and family. Women who have other children at home are likely to regard the hospital as a vacation hotel where they can saturate themselves with ease and luxury and tell everyone they could stay there for weeks.

But this is a first and second day delusion. They are kidding themselves.

Do you know what *really* happens? They get lonely. They want to go home. They become bored with hospital routine and anxious to have custody of the new baby. On the day of departure, almost invariably, the mother will arise early, dress, make herself as pretty as she can, then fidget around anxiously until her husband comes to take her home.

But as brief as the hospital time has come to be, a number of important steps are taken to prepare mother and baby for a good start together at home.

For example, if the woman is not going to nurse she may be given a combination of hormones that will help to turn off the mechanism that triggers the production of milk at about the third day.

These are female hormones that are now produced synthetically. If given with 24 hours of delivery they will help retard milk formation. They don't work every time. Sometimes there are cases of slight leakage, so the woman will have to wear breast bindings for a while until the flow stops. This it will do, for Nature finds no point in producing milk that isn't wanted.

The hormones given to suppress milk production can be overridden by the simple act of nursing. Let's say that the new mother decides that she wants to nurse, after all, but she has already been given the hormones. All she has to do is bring the baby to her breasts a few times, and she's back in business. The suckling action brings in the milk just about as copiously as though she had taken nothing.

Stopping the flow of milk, stimulating its production and maintaining an ample supply for a hungry baby have nothing at all to do with the size of the breasts. It's a natural assumption, I suppose, to conclude that a woman with ample breasts will produce a more abundant supply of milk than the one who may have done a lot of wishful thinking. Not necessarily so. It happens to be a stark medical fact that the major portion of tissue which leads to the coining of such words as "voluptuous" and "buxom" is nothing more elegant than fat. It may be impressively deployed, but it's still fat.

A small-breasted woman can have milk ducts that perform better than those of one who has always taken it for granted that her generous construction would obviously serve a nursing baby. I can't say that it runs as a rule that moderately endowed women nurse better, but it happens often enough for obstetricians to be able to give enthusiastic encouragement to them when they say they would love to nurse but are afraid they are too small.

A woman planning to breast feed will switch to a nursing bra rather than one designed for support alone. The chief advantage of the nursing bra is that it has trapdoors that expose the nipple area so that she doesn't have to take it off each time the baby must be fed. We in America tend to make a big fuss of modesty about breast feeding in public, but in most other countries it is an accepted function. With a nursing bra, plus an enlightened attitude, it is entirely possible for a woman to nurse discreetly without going off by herself. I know of a strikingly beautiful, poised young woman who brought her baby to a dinner table around which five guests were having coffee, and nursed it without causing the slightest flurry.

A nursing bra won't be necessary for two or three days after delivery, for milk production does not usually become copious enough to feed a baby until after the third day.

A nursing bra can hardly ever be of the right size because the size of the breasts keeps changing from one feeding to another. Some women are surprised, even shocked, to find that their breasts don't match after nursing. But at least they have the option of switching the baby from one to the other to equalize.

This is a much better deal than some women get during the pregnancy itself: one breast gets bigger than the other and *stays* that way. Brassiere makers have yet to cater to this unilateral oddity, probably because it's too complex. Which cup should be made bigger, the right or the left? And how much bigger?

Take comfort, you who are caught in this unequal bind; the condition is generally self-correcting whether you breast feed or not. Be confident that when it's all over, your margin of difference, if any, would have to be measured with calipers. In the casual appraisals so appreciated by women, no one is likely to know—including obstetricians.

Whether nursing or not, the *post-partum* patient continues to experience rapid reduction in the size of the uterus. It is quite astonishing that this organ, which has had to expand to 500 times its normal size to accommodate the baby, can return to its normal size so quickly. To the woman herself, it may seem a long time. But if she can remember how big it was, she can be patient about the time it takes to become unobtrusive again.

The same contractions that help the uterus to become obscure also tend to stifle the lingering minor bleeding and the flow of lochia. While in the hospital, the woman is checked every day to make sure that this part of the recovery process continues.

Blood tests are also made during the hospital stay to be certain that the patient is regaining her normal level of red cells. Every pregnant woman has a relative anemia; every woman who delivers loses blood. One of the most important reasons for staying in the hospital is to give her body time to replace the deficit in red cells, boosting the level of hemoglobin so that her circulation can carry oxygen to the various parts of her body more effectively.

If the woman is Rh-negative and has given birth to an Rh-positive baby, her blood will be re-checked for Rh antibodies. If she had none before this birth, there will not have been time for her to develop them. Even if this birth involved a blood exchange between her and the baby, an injection of Rhogam, given within 72 hours after birth, will stifle her body's normal immune response. The gamma globulin, which is rich in antibodies to Rh developed by Rh-negative donors, will attack and destroy any Rh-positive cells that happen to be circulating, so that her own system will not have to do it, and hence will remain free of any Rh threat to a future child.

But when an Rh-negative mother's *post-partum* blood test confirms that a titer of Rh antibodies is present, her doctor must assume that in this birth a blood transfer may have occurred which will boost her level of antibodies even higher. It would seem that an injection of Rhogam for such a woman would at least hold the level of antibodies down, but it doesn't. If there is any exchange, the next birth will pose a more serious Rh problem.

One *post-partum* protection against Rh response by Rhogam serves only that pregnancy. At each subsequent delivery the patient must be given another injection.

Altogether there are enough things to be done and to have done during the hospital stay to make a woman feel busy. And that includes the very practical resolution to get as much rest and sleep as she can to prepare herself for the rugged schedule she must meet when she gets home.

These four or five days are just as important to the baby. This is a tiny person whose energies are almost completely taken up by the arduous tasks of breathing and eating.

Why do newborns sleep so much?

Because they are pooped!

For an infant, a few minutes of being awake are enormously tiring. Consciousness requires rapid breathing, wiggling arms and legs, and hollering for attention. For someone who has literally never done a lick of work in its life, these actions are exhausting. Simply sucking a few ounces of milk out of breast or bottle is a major strain. So babies sleep because they are tired—so tired that they don't even have enough strength to hold their eyelids up.

When a baby is born, it becomes a pediatric patient. But it is first the responsibility of the obstetrician who delivers it. Moments later that responsibility is shared by the anesthetist in attendance; he must make sure that the child is breathing well and is capable of sustaining life on its own.

Later, the pediatrician will examine the baby and perform whatever services are necessary to insure its safety. If the mother has her own pediatrician, or wants the baby to be under the care of her family doctor, he will assume the medical responsibility.

There is one assignment, however, which remains with the obstetrician: circumcision of a boy. It is no longer to be taken for granted. Although the majority of physicians recommend it, recent research allows for argument that it may be unnecessary or "capricious" surgery. The case is well studied, but I still believe it to be a most beneficial procedure. However, I will not insist with parents who feel strongly that the penis should be left as delivered.

If the child is to be circumcised, the obstetrician will do it within the first few days, while the newborn's unique ability to shut out pain is still operative. The procedure is merely the cutting away of the foreskin so that it no longer covers the head of the penis.

We usually do this minor surgery on the second or third day in the hospital, so that it will be well on the way to healing by the time mother and baby are due to go home. The mother is shown how to take care of the slight wound when bathing or changing the baby.

There is not much controversy in my mind in the consideration of circumcision. It certainly makes care of the organ much easier for the mother while the baby is young, and the boy himself when he gets older. We can't say that hygienic neglect of the penis can cause cancer there. But we note rather solemnly that this form of cancer has never been reported in a circumcised male.

A delicate phase of what little debate is left is whether a circumcised man is more or less sensitive to the pleasures of sex as a result. It is obvious that a glans which is normally protected from stimuli by a foreskin will be more sensitive to contact when exposed, as it is during intercourse. But it is just as obvious that whatever a man

159

might lose in immediacy of response he will regain in duration of exposure.

It is probably difficult, or even impossible, for the mother of a newborn baby boy to consider the esthetics of her child as a grown man making love to a woman. Just take my word for it that such considerations have not been overlooked by medicine.

Therefore, for reasons of convenience and the prevention of medical and sanitary problems, I think every male child ought to be circumcised.

If the child's parents are Jewish, they should always be asked if they desire to have a ritual circumcision, performed by a rabbi. This may not be important to them, but I always like to make sure that there is consultation with grandparents or great-grandparents who might be offended if the affair makes no obeisance to religious tradition.

The parents themselves might not find the ritual important, but if it is meaningful to their more tradition-minded elders, it is a thoughtful gesture to defer to them.

I can't forget one little boy whose mother and father assured me that, though their parents were quite devout, they nevertheless wanted me to do the circumcision, rather than a rabbi. The afternoon after the surgery was done, I received a terribly irate call from the husband's mother, who told me I was unethical, insensitive, incompetent and irresponsible for having done medically what should have been done ritualistically.

I calmed her down and told her that I had discussed the circumcision with her son and his wife and had included telling them how important a ritual circumcision might be to grandparents. Then I said, "Before I did it, your daughter-in-law told me it would be all right."

There was a long pause, then the grandmother said: "Well, I didn't want him to marry her in the first place!"

In some hospitals it is the practice not to do circumcision unless or until the baby reaches a weight of at least six pounds. Almost all babies lose several ounces following delivery because they are constantly converting body tissue into the energy needed to sustain life.

The six-pound minimum for elective surgery is to prevent blood loss, which would make further inroads into the baby's modest reserves.

All babies weighing less than five pounds eight ounces are classified as premature, and are kept in the protected and controlled atmosphere of a nursery incubator. The term "premature" is no longer medically accurate, since it is a classification determined entirely by weight rather than by the number of days before term that the baby is born. It is true that most babies born early are small, but not all small babies are born early.

Because of intensive care and the oxygen-rich environment, borderline preemies often bounce back quickly and are ready to go home with their mother. But very small babies must stay behind when their mothers go home until they gain the weight and strength necessary to survive without problems.

It is generally true that the smaller the baby, the more complex are its troubles. This is because its margin of reserve energy and tissue is so narrow. A tiny baby has strength enough to take only a few ounces of nourishment before it falls asleep of exhaustion. Consequently, it is likely to gain weight only in fractions of ounces. But a baby of seven pounds or more has plenty of stored fat to draw upon during its first days of life. It can lose several ounces or even a pound or more, and still be able to make the voracious surge of appetite and energy output that can be expected in the second or third week of life.

Many young mothers are needlessly terrified when they get their new babies home and put them on the scale for the first time.

"He's lost seven ounces!"

They immediately leap to the conclusion that the hospital has grossly neglected the child, despite the fact that they, themselves, were probably responsible for most of the feedings.

Hospital nursery care includes many more assessments than gain or loss of weight. The amount and frequency of feedings are recorded; bowel and bladder activity are checked, the child is studied for its liveliness and response to stimuli such as snapping a finger on the sole of its foot; and its entire body is thoughtfully examined by people professionally alert to the slightest abnormality.

But of course the mother witnesses very little of this care because she's not there in the nursery. She can reassure herself this way: If *she's* getting good care herself, she can be sure her baby is getting even more attention.

In the short time mother and baby spend in the hospital they learn a good deal about each other—but not enough. At the dramatic moment when they are taken to the hospital door and the nurse places the baby in the mother's arms, there can easily be a flash of panic: "How in the world am I ever going to manage this?"

Try it. The first thing you may have to manage is how to get into the waiting automobile with a baby in your arms. It might make more sense to have somebody hand you the baby after you're seated, but mothers don't do this. Once the baby is put in their grasp, they don't like to yield, no matter if the ride home requires them to get into the bucket seat of an XKE Jaguar!

From first trial onward, parenthood is largely a matter of experimentation. You try things, and you either do well or badly. But babies happen to be highly durable people who are incredibly resistant to the effects of occasional bungling.

There is much to be done in bringing a new baby into the house. The shortened hospital stay requires the mother to make a very quick adjustment. One day she is surrounded by all kinds of professional help in the care of her baby, and on the next she suddenly finds herself in sole command.

This is why it has become a desirable luxury to have some sort of skilled, professional person at home for a week or so. It is not because the new mother is too debilitated from her delivery, for in most cases she's not. Modern obstetrical practice has eliminated much of the bodily wear and tear that earlier women withstood as a matter of course.

But there is a welter of things for a new mother to do, many of which she may never have had to do before. Ideally, she ought to be able to learn her new trade calmly, without facing a new crisis every hour or so. She needs someone with her for help and company.

But the assistant ought not to be a family relation. Well-meaning relatives can somehow create crisis the way heat produces popcorn. Tensions in this period tend to run high, but they can often be set in balance by the presence of someone who is there to help but not in a position to be critical or to be criticized.

The transition to life at home may be made more acute by

something most maternity patients feel, but few ever mention. The man upon whom so much depended, and who paid them such close professional attention—the obstetrician—seems to have dropped them entirely.

He hasn't, really. It is just that his services are being required by women who need them now as urgently as you did when you went into labor. The routine of maternity wards is such that a *post-partum* patient can be carefully monitored without constant attention from her physician; a daily visit may be all that is required. Your doctor may not even examine you before your departure for home unless there is some special reason why he should.

After leaving his custody to return home, the woman realizes there is now no further reason to telephone the doctor, as there was during the last weeks before delivery when she was one of his special considerations. Now there are six weeks ahead before she will return for a checkup. So the intensely close relationship is over, for now. Many women feel this loss quite strongly, especially during those minor frustrations that occur in coping with a new baby. Shrug this off; take my word for it that an obstetrician would be clumsy with a bottle and useless with a diaper anyway.

It is a rare female who finds she is able to take up her new duties joyfully and efficiently from the start. Those who have help for the first week or two enjoy the bonus of being able to select which chores they'll do themselves, and how fast they'll work toward carrying the entire load.

So far as physical capacity is concerned, you are probably capable of doing as much as you please, but don't press it. Sleep is nearly as important to you as it is to your baby. You may find yourself willing to take a nap or a rest at a time when the baby sleeps. But if you don't feel fatigue, you may safely undertake just about any household activity without feeling that you are still too fragile for it.

The healing process will continue for several weeks. Muscles and organs that took the strains and stresses of delivery will repair themselves, and the uterus will continue to reduce itself to a size nearly as small as it was before conception.

Normal physical activity helps the processes of repair by stimulating blood circulation and increasing the respiration rate. But don't get jumpy about starting gymnastic exercise; it would be unwise until after your six-weeks checkup. You have not yet passed the point of vulnerability to damage from straining tissue that is still undergoing recovery. Besides, your efforts to tighten and tone up those tummy muscles will be futile until the uterus shrinks back enough so that it won't press on them, and undo anything you might accomplish.

Though normal activity is encouraged, pace is its key. Try to make your motions deliberate. If the telephone rings, avoid the impulse reaction. Anyone who really must speak to you will stay on the line until the bell sounds ten times; if you move toward the phone slowly and casually, you will still get there on the fourth or fifth ring.

The same applies when the baby begins to stir. Instead of leaping up, take a moment to analyze the nature of the crying. You will find that an important skill of motherhood is learning from a baby's sound how urgent is its message.

Do you have stairs in your home? Here's a precept: Every trip over the stairs will do you some good, but only if you don't trip over the stairs.

Take your time. Especially in those moments when you feel there is no time to take.

There is another activity to be resumed following a woman's return from having a baby: intercourse with her husband. She will surely have qualms about it for a while because she has been tender and sore in that area. But many women needlessly fear the possibility of pain long after they have healed, and thereby cause themselves and their husbands unnecessary grief and frustration.

Most doctors will advise that intercourse not be resumed until after the six-weeks checkup. There is always the possibility that early intercourse might introduce infection, or cause damage to tissues that are not completely healed. This is sound medical advice, but we are not surprised when it isn't strictly followed.

Some women fear that they will be vulnerable to tearing because an incision was made in the vagina. This is true only if relations are attempted too early. But once the healing is complete the tissue is as strong as it ever was. In fact, in many cases of virginal women who became pregnant shortly after marriage, intercourse proved to be much more pleasurable after delivery than it was before.

Be assured also that when your doctor is stitching you up

following delivery, he is not altogether occupied by the immediate surgical business. He is fully aware of the fact that his arrangement of stitches will later have an important bearing on the degree of pleasure to be derived by both husband and wife. The surgery calls for mere skill; the style demands art, and any obstetrician, if he's candid enough, will acknowledge his pride in this art.

By the time six weeks have passed, the sutures will have been absorbed by the body and inflammation or tenderness will have disappeared from the sensitive tissue. When the doctor verifies by examination that all is well, the woman need have no fears about the resumption of love-making. Surely she must understand that this has been a long abstinence from intercourse, just as her husband must understand that she will require special tenderness and care as they resume.

There is more to be said on this subject, yet I do so with hesitancy that I am sure would be shared by most obstetricians. For in this field we often see an unhappy aspect of the function of sex in marriage.

When I find by examination that it is safe for a woman to resume her sex life, I like to say to her, "I now pronounce you man and wife." It may be a corny line, but many women respond with a smile that tells me they are pleased to be back in condition for the giving and receiving of love. Or there may be a grin that suggests my pronouncement wasn't necessary.

Many others, however, make a different response:

"Don't you dare tell my husband!"

Sometimes there's a note of jest, sometimes I know it is said in dead earnest. Either way, I cannot help but suspect that all is not well in their physical relations with their mates. A reliable study finds that some 85 per cent of married couples in America are not well adjusted sexually. We who so often hear negative reactions toward the resumption of sex can easily believe that figure.

Most people think that the province of obstetrics is the delivery of babies, not their conception. Yet if we are responsible for the fitness of women to bear children, that fitness includes their receptivity to the means by which babies are begun.

Sex is a function of the body. As in any part of the body, malfunction is a medical problem. But it is one which society's canons of privacy have made none of a doctor's business unless and until his service is sought.

Even psychiatrists find themselves severely limited in matters of sex advice and treatment. The result is that we have a rampant, untreated disease against which no medical attack can be made because so many pretend the disease does not exist.

If a doctor were to detect diabetes in a patient and fail to treat it until the woman acknowledged that she had the disease, he would be guilty of gross neglect.

Yet again and again, we see the affliction of negative attitude toward sex, and we can say nothing.

But sound advice is available for a woman who finds herself unhappy on being told she can make love again. Furthermore, I believe this advice to be an integral part of responsible obstetrical practice. It is this:

Any woman who wishes to bear other children, or to serve well in motherhood for those she already has, must have complete health, including health of her mind. A child conceived without enthusiasm is not likely to be carried with glee. Just as strong desire can create a false pregnancy, so can aversion to sex cause trouble in a true pregnancy.

Therefore I would solemnly suggest that any woman who is unhappy when told she can resume intercourse should tell her doctor exactly that. He has several ways in which he might be able to help.

For example, he might detect that some unpleasant phase of her pregnancy is the cause. He may help her overcome any physical impediment to good sex, such as painful intercourse. Or he might suggest psychiatric or psychological treatment to help her achieve a healthy and responsive attitude.

But this assistance and advice should be asked for. I believe a physician ought to open his door for you. He might say casually, "Do you want to talk about it?" But whether he does or not, if you have the slightest thought that your own well-being might be improved by ridding yourself of reservations about sex, make yourself bring it up now. For this *is* a proper subject in obstetrics.

Another event that the new mother anticipates is the return of her normal menstrual cycle. This will probably occur some time between two weeks and three months after confinement. When the first period is delayed a woman is apt to suspect that she has conceived again. She probably hasn't. Here we can shoot down another old wives' tale that says if a woman is not nursing and has resumed relations with her husband she will conceive more readily than ever. Absolutely untrue.

A woman is actually *less* likely to conceive because she is less likely to ovulate, and less likely to have created a receptive atmosphere inside her uterus.

The only true part of the tale is that breast feeding does have a contraceptive effect. But nursing a baby is far from foolproof as a method of birth control. And after 11 months, it is completely unreliable.

If the first period has not occurred by the time of the six-weeks visit, and the woman, nursing or not, wishes to practice some form of birth control, she can be provided with a method then, rather than wait for the first period. This is because true menstruation does not take place until 14 days after an ovum has been released; since a woman has no reliable way of knowing when she will release that first, receptive egg, she will not be aware that her body has become ready to conceive.

The first period itself may be extremely heavy, with many clots and a flow that is longer than usual. This tends to throw some women into a panic. It won't if you know that such a flow is to be expected.

However, if the flow seems to be too copious for too long a time, a woman should, of course, inform her doctor. He may put her on a course of ergotrate and have her place ice bags on her abdomen. These steps will usually stem the flow. Very rarely the woman may have to be brought into the hospital for treatment of an excessive first period.

It is instinctively maternal for a woman to be so preoccupied with her baby that she is less aware of the doings inside her own body. This is fortunate, for most women recover nicely, resume their menstrual cycle, and carry on as before.

Well—not quite as before. For now they'll spend a lot of time digging up baby sitters.

SIX WEEKS CHECKUP

it's been grand, really!

Notice to mothers: bringing a baby to an obstetrician's office is utterly unnecessary, except when contained in the original package. Leave it at home—please!

Is there a sound reason for a six-weeks checkup?

I believe this visit to be so important to the mother's health, as do most obstetricians, that I make it clear in the discussion of fee that the *post-partum* examination is included. Further, if a patient doesn't call me for an appointment at about that time, I will have someone call to remind her that she is due.

The most compelling reason for examination following delivery is to make an appraisal of the cervix. This organ is a common site for the development of cancer in a woman. But it happens to be an accessible organ, which means that examination can anticipate conditions favorable for malignant growth, and steps can be taken to prevent it.

Medicine does not yet know precisely what causes cancer, but we have learned many things about the conditions under which it can get started. For example, we know that a site where there is a long-standing inflammation can eventually become malignant.

It is inevitable that a full-term cervix will tear as the baby passes through it, causing lacerations. Ordinarily these lacerations will heal following delivery. They leave their mark in the form of a familiar "fish-mouth" scar. When the healing is complete, the scar serves only to indicate that the woman has had a child, and that the cervix has repaired itself.

But if there is a partial failure in the healing process, the laceration can remain continually inflamed. If neglected or undiscovered, such an inflammation can ultimately cause trouble.

Because the cervix is so accessible, the once devastating ravages of cancer there have been brought under excellent medical control. The only cases we are likely to see now are those in which there was no regular medical scrutiny of the site.

Detection of a potentially dangerous cervical condition is determined by a microscopic examination. Sloughed-off cells, taken from the cervix by swab, are studied for certain shapes, formation and cellular structure. Experienced pathologists can recognize these as potentially malignant.

This is a marvelous advantage; we can detect and treat the pre-malignant condition long before it develops into actual cancer, and we can do so by a lead time of three to 11 years.

The technique is the now famous Pap smear, named for Dr. George Papanicolaou, the gynecologist who devised it in 1933. It is our most dependable method of screening for cancer. Every woman, whether she has had no children or 15 children should have the Pap smear test done regularly throughout her lifetime.

The doctor does not rely entirely on the Pap test in the *post-partum* checkup. When he can see that there are areas of inflammation in the cervix he can treat them directly by the use of heat, or cautery, and even a newer method, freezing or cryosurgery. This probably sounds terrifying, but don't worry about it; the cervix happens to be an organ that is virtually insensitive to pain.

The doctor will also examine the episiotomy scar for good repair, and check for the presence of any growths, enlargements or other abnormalities in the female organs.

This is also the proper time for discussion of a method of birth control, if it is desired. Most modern women hope for some sort of respite from conception, even if it is to be the rhythm method. The religious considerations must be entirely your own; your doctor's only function is to advise which method he feels is best for your particular circumstances.

If the choice is to be the Intrauterine Device (IUD), the doctor can install it now. Some clinics are experimenting with insertion of the

IUD on the fourth day after delivery, but results have not been entirely encouraging. The cervix is still quite open and the device tends to drop out.

Installation at the six weeks visit is a bit more difficult, but protection against conception is better. When properly placed in a uterus contracted down to its normal size, the device is quite reliable. The wearer herself can check on its continuing presence by feeling in her vagina for the nylon strand attached to it and extending downward through the cervix.

The following may sound like a recital of broad areas of ignorance in female biology, but we don't yet know exactly how the IUD works. The fact that it makes contact with the walls of the uterus, thereby causing a mild superficial inflammation, suggests that it might prevent a fertilized egg from implanting. Or its mere presence as a foreign object inside the uterus might trigger the woman's expulsive responses so that any conception which comes down is doomed to ejection. There is also some indication that the presence of the IUD somehow affects the sperm, perhaps frustrating its efforts to swim toward the waiting egg.

However the IUD functions, it is a dependable contraceptive when it is correctly in place. But it can be improperly installed, and it can be dislodged. This is why the figures on the efficiency of the IUD are somewhat less than 100 per cent. There is also a body of evidence being gathered that shows that an increased number of pelvic inflammations are associated with IUD's, plus an increased number of tubal pregnancies. So you see, any method, however expedient, has its drawbacks.

Some women may choose to return to the diaphragm, though recent evidence suggests this is less dependable. Studies indicate that in some women the sexual climax is accompanied by a ballooning of the upper vagina. This permits the diaphragm to float out of contact with surrounding tissues. Unless adequate spermicidal foam or jelly is present, sperm can get past the barrier and into the uterus.

If the diaphragm is to be used, the doctor can measure to be sure that the original size worn is still correct, as it probably is.

The diaphragm, the IUD, contraceptive jelly and foam, and the condom worn by the husband are forms of contraception that serve with varying degrees of assurance. The rhythm method is as notable for its failures as for its successes.

The most effective method of birth control known is the contraceptive pill. Taken correctly—and I mean exactly according to directions—it is virtually a perfect contraceptive. There have been human errors—a woman who forgets a pill, or who confuses her dates—but the pill itself is foolproof.

But is it safe?

Probably. There is some statistical indication that there may be hazards for certain women who take it. Thus far the danger remains only statistical, however. It can be seen that among large numbers of women who have taken the pill, there is a higher incidence of thrombophlebitis, the same clotting condition we seek to avoid by having a woman get up and walk a little shortly after delivery. The figures also show slightly more pulmonary embolism, which is a clotting condition affecting the lungs; and cerebro-vascular accidents, best known as strokes.

This does NOT mean that when a patient suffers one of these conditions it can necessarily be blamed upon having taken the pill. It might mean—and much more research is necessary to confirm this—that a woman's susceptibility to any of these threats may be increased by the use of the pill.

There are disadvantages to the pill which may influence a woman's desire to use it. Because it is a steroid drug, it tends to make the body retain fluids, just as the estrogen of pregnancy does. This means you may have slightly swollen fingers and ankles, a bloated feeling, and perhaps headaches and blurring of vision.

The breasts may enlarge as they did in pregnancy, and the areolae of the nipples may darken. Very susceptible women also develop cloasma, the mask of pregnancy, as a result of taking the pill.

Merely by withdrawing from it, these symptoms can be made to disappear. Most women find them no more than bothersome, at worst. Sometimes such symptoms are relieved by changing from one form of the pill to another. A few women decide that the absolute security of the pill is not worth the misery it causes them, so they try some other method of contraception.

Formerly there were two principal types of pill that enjoyed popularity. One was called "sequential." For the first 15 days, the woman took a pill containing estrogen as its only hormone. For the next five days she took one which combined estrogen with another hormone, progesterone. This type of pill is off the market, unavailable.

The type of pill most commonly used now is called "combined," because it contains both estrogen and progesterone, and is taken daily for 20 or 21 days. The woman then takes no hormones for a week, and resumes taking the combined form again. For convenience, several manufacturers of contraceptive pills supply 28 tablets, to be taken one per day every day, including the fourth week. But the last seven pills contain no medication; they are merely a convenience toward keeping dates straight.

What is the effect of these two components? Estrogen by itself will prevent ovulation, but if taken alone for a protracted period, will cause nausea and vomiting. When balanced by the presence of progesterone, these symptoms are suppressed.

Progesterone taken by itself can prohibit conception without preventing ovulation, though we are not yet sure how the effect is accomplished. The evidence strongly suggests that progesterone alters the chemistry of the cervical mucus in such a way that sperm cannot survive its passage. There is also the possibility that progesterone changes the character of the temporary lining in the uterus so that if a fertilized ovum does arrive from the fallopian tube, it is unable to implant itself on the uterine wall, and so is eventually sloughed out.

If there is a villain in the contraceptive pill it is probably the estrogen, and research efforts are already well advanced toward eliminating it. In fact, the pill which has made an international reputation for itself as the most effective method of birth control ever devised, is probably now in the twilight of its usage.

What seems to lie ahead is a mini-dose of progesterone daily, either by mouth or by implantation of a device just under the skin in some inconspicuous place on the body. The implanted container will release just enough progesterone each day to prevent a favorable climate for conception, and will contain enough of the material to last for many months.

If the woman bearing such a device decides she would like to become pregnant again, her doctor will simply remove it, and in a few days the suppressive effect of the hormone will be gone, and she will soon revert to her normal, receptive condition.

In the United States, the pill, the IUD, foam and other methods are largely a matter of convenience. Among women of more or less affluent means, they permit the spacing of babies. But in most of the world these methods of contraception become a matter of life and death. For populations already in poverty must achieve control over their birth rates, or they face mass starvation. This is why a monumental effort is being made to provide effective programs for distribution of contraceptive equipment among people whose birth rates literally threaten their continued existence.

But the population explosion is likely to be far afield from the consideration of an American woman who has just had a baby and would like a year or so for a breather before she starts another. For her I would recommend the pill.

The obstetrician offering the pill to a patient can write the prescription so it will last as long as he chooses. Many of us write them for only six months, because we want the woman to come back for examination. This is because the pill is comparatively new, and because it can cause side effects. We want to be sure that no side effects are developing untended. A woman with a tendency toward fibroid tumors, for example, may show on examination that the pill has accelerated their growth.

But even though a prescription is written only for a fixed period of time, the pills have become available just about willy-nilly. This is surely a contributing reason for the statistics on unpleasant and ominous side effects.

Under scrupulous control, with the user of the pill subject to regular medical attention, I feel that the pill is safe. But we still find people who will overdose themselves with as benevolent a medication as aspirin. So it is not surprising that we have cases in which long-term unsupervised taking of the contraceptive pill results in medical problems.

Ideally, this method of birth control should be a gentle regulation of natural processes. Ultimately it will be. It is very close to that goal now. But it is important that any user of these hormones have some sound understanding of what is going on.

When you take a contraceptive pill that contains estrogen, ovulation is prevented. Therefore true menstruation, by definition, does not take place. For menstruation is uterine bleeding that follows ovulation by two weeks. It is "the funeral dirge of a disappointed and dejected egg." When an ovum has no rendezvous with a sperm, it deteriorates and is absorbed in body fluids. Meanwhile, down in the uterus, an entirely new lining—the endometrium—has developed for the sole purpose of receiving a fertilized egg if it should arrive. If it does not, the body sloughs off the new membrane, exposing small blood vessels which break and bleed in the process. This is the material of menstruation.

The tissue grown to line the uterus is altered by the presence of the progesterone in the pill, enough so that it becomes unsuitable for the implantation of a fertilized egg. But the estrogen prevents ovulation, so no conception can take place. Both phases of the cycle are thus inhibited, therefore the normal cycle is incomplete. This is the reason that the period of a woman on the pill is likely to be shorter and less copious. First of all, there is no ovum, and second, the uterine lining to be disposed of was not complete.

The abbreviated period worries some women terribly, because they think that the reduced flow can only mean that they are pregnant. Actually, the moderate, brief menses is a bonus convenience that inevitably must result from the bodily effects of taking the pill.

What happens if ovulation is suppressed for a very long time by the use of the pill—say for years? We don't know, because the pill hasn't been around long enough. Some doctors ask their patients to withdraw from the pill for a month or so after taking it for 18 months. They want to allow a full, normal menstrual cycle to take place. This is a commendable medical precaution, but I think that when the pill has had a longer record of performance, it will prove unnecessary.

We have talked about going on the pill. What happens when a woman goes off of it?

We know that when a woman stops taking the pill, her first period is likely to be considerably delayed; it will probably occur 40 to 45 days after she stops.

Once again, of course, she'll probably think that she is pregnant. But if she has taken reasonable precautions during her period of abstinence from the pill, she probably will not have conceived.

The long time lapse is usually creditable to the wonderfully adaptive talent of Nature, returning conditions to normal.

When Nature is *ab*normal, this unique medication can help bring it into line. In the case of a woman who has a history of radically shifting menstrual cycles, the pill will most often help to produce a more regular period. Why? Because the taking of the pill inhibits uterine bleeding. When the pill is withdrawn, the woman will bleed.

Another surprising bonus of the pill is its ability to relieve menstrual discomfort. A woman who has experienced cramps during her normal period will usually find that they are relieved by the pill. This is consistent with the reduced activity the pill's ingredients cause—no ovulation, limited development of the endometrium, lessened bleeding.

Currently, there is some concern that the pill may repress the capacity for a woman to conceive after she stops taking it. This is because some women who have relinquished its protection report that they have difficulty in getting pregnant. Does this mean that the pill dampens reproductive capacities? Probably not. For included among former pill-users whose fertility seems impaired are those whose fertility has never been fairly tested. These are women who started taking the pill as soon as they became eligible for intercourse. We know that such a group must contain a certain percentage of women for whom conception would have been difficult anyway. What we don't know is how many of them may be blaming a natural infertility on the fact that they took the pill.

Therefore, the woman returning to her doctor following delivery and wishing to defer another pregnancy need not necessarily be concerned that she might be jeopardizing her ability to bear children by the use of the pill. We know that these hormones can cause a temporary upset in the return of the normal cycle, but there is nothing in the record to prove that they might disturb natural fertility.

Suppose a woman wants to have several more babies, conveniently spaced? How much of a toll does each sequence of pregnancy, labor and delivery take on her body?

Because obstetrics has become as modern as a Saturn V rocket, women can now carry their children with less effort, labor toward their delivery with less pain, and deliver them with reduced cost to their bodies.

In the days when labor was allowed to proceed for a very long time—beyond 18 to 24 hours—terrible strains were imposed, not only upon the organs directly involved in childbirth, but also upon bladder, rectum and other adjacent tissues. Gynecologists must still devote much of their time to repair of such damage among older women who labored so hard and so long to deliver their babies.

The four or five extra hours that were necessary to expel an unusually large or poorly positioned baby required, in later years, extensive plastic surgery in the pelvis, to say nothing of the long period of discomfort and pain usually endured before the surgery was done.

But these days we will not let a woman labor so long. We use low forceps to negotiate a baby's head through a difficult passage. Episiotomy reduces the resistance against which the mother's powers must push. Benign anesthesia eliminates the pain that can distort the efficiency of her own delivery prowess. The modern woman can come out of the birth experience with far more reserve energy and far less physical damage.

From all reasonable observations of the human species, we deduce that it should be natural and joyful for a man and a woman to produce proof of their own worth in the intended order of this universe—reproduction, in the form of offspring who carry on with their own particular talents and inclinations. The process is hazardous, but the dangers contribute to the divine excitement. Parenthood is marked by strain, uncertainty and challenge. Consequently, when all goes well, the reward is glorious.

And through it all there is always the sense of miracle and wonder. It is absolutely stupefying that the complex elements of pursuit, love-making, gestation, labor, and delivery can ultimately produce something as incredibly perfect as a baby, insistently bent upon thriving and growing to maturity.

Humans are the only living creatures upon this earth who are capable of understanding the glory of their own reproduction. This is, perhaps, the ultimate privilege of having the only mind, among all known animal species, that is sophisticated enough to perceive its own existence.

Women understand this intuitively, for it is they who bear our babies. Obstetricians share it, because they are privileged to assist.

Congratulations on your new baby, madam!

And, although it has been done before, nobody in all of history has done it quite the way you did.

INDEX